Understanding   Your   Disease

THE
SYMBOLIC
MESSAGE OF
ILLNESS

*An Adventure in
Knowing Yourself*

Calin V. Pop, MD

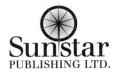

Sunstar
PUBLISHING LTD.

THE SYMBOLIC MESSAGE OF ILLNESS
by Calin V. Pop, MD

©1999
United States Copyright
Sunstar Publishing, Ltd.
116 North Court Street
Fairfield, Iowa 52556

Cover Design: **Irene Archer**
Editor: **Isabel Hubert**
Layout & Design: **Sharon A. Dunn**

LCCN: **96-69529**
ISBN: **1-887472-16-9**

If you are unable to order this book from your local bookseller,
you may order directly from the publisher. Quantity discounts
for organizations are available. Call toll free: **(800) 532-4734**.

This material has been written and published solely for educational purposes.

*The author of this book does not dispense medical advice nor prescribe the
use of any technique as a form of treatment for physical or medical problems
without the advice of a physician, either directly or indirectly. The intent of
the author is only to offer information of a general nature to help you in your
quest for physical fitness and good health. In the event that you use any of the
information in this book for yourself, which is your constitutional right,
the author and the publisher assume no responsibility for your actions.*

*The author and publisher shall have neither liability or responsibility
to any person or entity with respect to any loss, damage or injury
caused or alleged to be caused directly or indirectly by
the information contained in this book.*

Readers interested in obtaining further information
on the subject matter of this book are invited to correspond with:

The Secretary, Sunstar Publishing, Ltd.
116 North Court Street, Fairfield, Iowa 52556

For more Sunstar Books, visit: *http://www.newagepage.com*

❖ ❖ ❖

"My family doesn't know that I can fly," she said.
"I don't have to tell them, do I?"

"When it is time for them to know,
you will not have to tell them."

❖ ❖ ❖

ACKNOWLEDGMENTS

I would like to acknowledge the many wonderful authors who helped me crystallize my ideas.

It is my opinion that when we read or hear something that touches our heart, we need to appreciate that message for its value, regardless of its source. Whether knowledge comes from the highest authority in the field or from the homeless at the corner of the street, its intrinsic value remains the same. It is our heart that speaks through their mouth. We would not be able to appreciate someone else's opinion unless that opinion has already been located in ourselves, even though it may have been hidden and ignored. We always need to resonate with an idea in order to perceive it. The time has come to focus on the message, not on who said it. Once we get beyond judging our sources, we can accept or reject ideas based on their true, intrinsic value.

For these reasons, there will be no sources listed after quotations, nor will a strict reference be kept. Even my name is not important. So, for accuracy and in order to eliminate the footnotes which I believe are annoying, the sources of many quotes will be in the bibliography at the end of the book. There the reader can access them, preferably **after** he or she has made a decision whether to accept the point of view or not. I have to admit that there are some sources of quotes and other inspirations that I don't remember any more.

However, I hereby offer my acknowledgements, gratitude and deep appreciation to all.

TABLE OF CONTENTS

LIST OF FIGURES, TABLES AND CHARTS

Figures:

Tables:

Charts:

INTRODUCTION

The purpose of this book is to help you become more aware.
My primary goal is to offer my reader an awakening tool for a new awareness and a new understanding. This understanding can be applied in many ways in daily life. Health care treatments and techniques abound, but too often they end up being nothing more than "crutches," not solving the actual problem. People are now ready for something more profound than that. I believe that the answer lies not in yet another healing modality, but in a change of awareness, a replacement of a habit, and a new way of living life.

This book was written for everyone; medical knowledge is not required. I intend to keep the information simple and easy to understand at an intuitive level. It is up to you how much you want to absorb, how much you grow or evolve. There are no quotas or time limits. Everybody grows in his own way, time and style. You can choose and, in fact, you WILL choose the lessons that will benefit you the most, either consciously or not. There is no set pace, there are no outside goals. Only you, the reader, can decide how much you need to understand or how far you should go in this adventure. Trust that the ideas you are attracted to explore and understand further are the ones most appropriate for you. You may jump ahead and read what seems attractive to you, but you will probably benefit more from enjoying this journey in a step-by-step fashion. Step-by-step is the way I myself arrived at this understanding, over the course of several years. Let me tell you how it happened:

One day I was asked to give a seminar. A small chart was given to me with the intention that it might be of some help. It was a Chinese symbolic correlation table (**Chart 1**) that you may find on pages 34 and 35. I became intrigued by the unusual relationships between human organs and other elements on the chart. Medically, the chart did not make sense, but then I realized that the connecting element was symbolic. I started to read more about symbols, and gradually came to understand more about the symbolic mirroring concept. This led to a chain reaction in self discovery. As I became more aware of the mechanics of my own inner workings, curious circumstances began happening to me: I was dealing with relationship problems at the time, and was ordered to do a rotation in cardiology. It seemed interesting that my symbolically "aching heart" was surrounded by heart disease. Was this a coincidence? Within a month I learned that I had to let go of some preconceived notions of mine and found myself doing a rotation in kidney disease. Was it coincidental that the kidneys also have to do with letting go? Also, just when I wasn't willing to accept higher aspects of myself, I found it difficult to explain higher meanings of disease to patients who were not yet ready to accept such explanations. Was this coincidental too? I decided to investigate this further.

I noticed that I had intensive care unit rotation when I had severe difficulties accepting myself. Whatever my own internal state, the patients seemed to be mirroring an aspect of it. When I was ready for a new set of experiences, they showed up – seemingly out of the blue, but with perfect timing. The connections were irrefutable. I learned to identify my own problems by paying attention to the world around me. I caught myself coughing and catching colds in response to messages that I didn't like. It was often challenging and humbling to face my problems, swallow my pride and learn my lessons. The human ego doesn't easily accept the fact that it needs to shape up and change. However, I learned that, just as we catch flies with honey, not vinegar, in the same way we heal our body by respecting its disease symptoms, not by suppressing them. The rewards of being open made it all worthwhile. All these were valued experiences that helped me become a stronger, more self-aware person.

The symbolic approach to disease may reveal challenging concepts to you, the reader, as well. We may perceive these challenges as "negative" because they represent our weaknesses or internal conflicts. These aspects are brought to the surface of our consciousness in order to be healed; there is no need for blame. For example, if you have arthritis, you will most likely take issue with the chapters about arthritis. This is a signal for you to pay close attention, because there lies the key for your healing. Remember that all great discoveries ultimately originate from a willingness to take the chance of not being right.

In order to solve any problem we first need to be aware of it. Only then can we *do* something about it. However, these two steps – to awareness and then to healing – are not exclusive or unique. There are many ways to awareness and many ways to healing. This book was designed to offer only one method to enhance your awareness. The healing will flow naturally from awareness when the time is right.

This book offers you a system of knowledge, nothing more. There is no need for me to "stand behind" it; there is no need for anyone to impose their point of view upon others. The ideas presented here are not a matter of true or false, right or wrong; they are more like your left hand that does not need to fight your right hand. Both hands constitute parts of a greater whole – your body. If one hand is of equal value to the other, then it doesn't really matter which one is chosen to fly a kite. It becomes a question of personal preference and cooperation, rather than competition.

This book is not rejecting other methods leading to awareness or labeling them as "better" or "worse." Also, it does not recommend one healing method over another; they ultimately are as good or as bad as we believe them to be. In fact, this book is not designed to address or promote healing modalities themselves. They will be the subject of another book.

In a way, this book is a rough re-writing of medicine from a symbolic perspective. Because I am only one person, I have not yet symbolically matched in a few years what the medical world did in several centuries. This is why not all details of disease symbolism will be explained here.

Some may wonder why I'm not using a more scientific method. Science is a way – fashionable nowadays – of seeing and understanding the world based on "proving." This method has opened us to a wonderful set of experiences, especially in the past century.

Science says, "Prove it and we will believe it." Other methods suggest that we only experience what we believe is possible and offer a different approach: "Believe it and then it will prove itself." In other words, we create our own experiences based on our knowledge and expectations, not the other way around. This approach can be found in modern quantum physics as well as in ancient scriptural texts. It is not better or worse, just different, and it may lead us to an equally wonderful set of experiences. When we are open to both sets, it is like being adept at using both the right and left hand; our universe expands and we have more choices – more freedom.

Somebody once said, "Action comes from belief, not the other way around, because belief is much deeper." Paradigms (points of view) are created and adopted; they can never be proven. If indeed we create realities through our focus, then we can build new realities simply by changing our focus – by consciously placing our attention in different directions. All of a sudden there is nothing to prove, because our attention is a matter of choice and acceptance, rather than proving. We are now back to, but far beyond, religion. The circle is closing.

Ultimately, "every truth is a seed within a bigger truth," so we need to practice being open to bigger truths.

If, after reading this book, you understand why you may have a headache or feel inspired to explore why you cough so often, then this book fulfilled its purpose. I understand that it might be difficult for many to accept that illness may have a serving purpose, but it is all a matter of raising our perspective. Illness can be a tremendous source of growth and wisdom, whether this is consciously acknowledged or not.

This book is not intended to promote one type of traditional or nontraditional approach over another. These ideas are not taken from the traditional Chinese medicine and also are not a compilation of different sources, even though I drew inspiration from many of them. Of course, there are many authors and readings that shaped my ideas over the years, but those were filtered through my beliefs and experience. Some basic concepts are taken from those wonderful materials listed in the bibliography, but most of this book is original. The Chinese concepts were only used in **Part II**, for the particular purpose of exemplifying a symbolic connection between different concepts.

Symbols can be powerful tools in helping us understand human nature and the process of illness. Instead of alienating us from our nature, symbols bring back openness, harmony, and spirituality. They draw us together to enhance our connection with nature and human consciousness. They shine a light into a shady corner and the darkness will disappear. When we shine open-minded awareness into an inner disturbance it will transform into positive, empowering qualities.

I now wish you fun and delight in this adventure of knowing yourself.

Part I

SYMBOLS

❖ ❖ ❖

"The only thing that shapes the Universe is your own conception of it."

❖ ❖ ❖

SYMBOLS

Part I of this book explores what a symbol is and how it can help you understand the reality around you. In **Part II**, we will analyze different organs, body parts and systems from a symbolic perspective. **Chart 1** *(Five Phase Correspondences)* on pages 34 and 35 will serve as a basis for discussion and further understanding of the symbols. In **Part III**, I outline a symbolic approach to disease and briefly analyze different symptoms. Some common illnesses will be approached here in order to make the process more understandable. **Part IV** describes cells and perception and **Part V**, the last and largest part, contains more detailed symbolic interpretations of some of the most common diseases. Many of them contain examples similar to case histories that will reinforce the more abstract descriptions of disease.

We may wonder why an unfamiliar place feels familiar or why we feel an instant attraction to someone we never met before. Why does holding hands make us feel safe and secure? Did we ever think about why Christmas carols put us in the Christmas spirit? These mechanics have to do with symbols. All of the above

examples – indeed all life events – are filled with symbolic implications that may trigger different emotional responses in us.

What is a Symbol?

The word symbol means "to bring together" and "to inte-
grate." Think of the word symbol as "same bowl," as if certain
things were being placed into the same bowl. Symbol formation
is an ongoing internal process of integrating life experiences
within our subconscious mind. We are continuously correlating
new experiences with old ones, whether they are linked in time
and space or appear separated. For example the symbol of a
cross may bring together joy and sorrow, duality and integration,
religious and mundane experiences ... in actuality, it brings all
these meanings together.

How Do Symbols Work?

Symbols may have hundreds of meanings that blend together
harmoniously and merge into new interpretations as often as
needed. It is not important nor possible to know them all or
bring them all to a conscious level, but they burst to the
conscious surface in the form of emotions, knowings and understandings. The whole complexity of meanings and representations is not accessed by the conscious mind; this would be
overload. For example, if someone wants to hear a certain piece
of news in a room full of different radio stations, they become
automatically oblivious to the sound of other stations nearby.
Yet, the other stations are blasting, and they can choose to
become aware of it at any moment.

In the same way, the whole complexity of symbol meanings is
never accessed by the conscious mind. All meanings are subconsciously processed, then the conscious mind "attunes" only to
the group of meanings that we need at a given time, constantly
adjusting the wave length as necessary. We may choose to ignore

the message, but it is there. By doing this, we may deny ourselves a set of experiences. If we choose something, it is not to be considered good or bad, it is after all just what we want to listen to at that point in time. If we want the silence, we just choose to ignore the message. If we want to access the rock station or the country station, we then attune to a specific frequency of transmission in order to have that specific experience. We may change it or we may keep it. My rock music is not any better or worse than the country music (some people may disagree here). It is not a question of good or bad, it is just what we want, need and like. However, the music is being transmitted all the times.

We are all here to experience different things in life in order to advance on our spiritual path. Since all individuals are different, we all tend to attune to different meanings of the same symbol. Some people may think of money as evil, while others see it as a wonderful thing. We usually find similar interpretations in people who have similar life experiences. Bankers, for example, perceive the money symbol in similar ways, which are probably different from the way homeless people may perceive it.

Symbols and Signs

Think about a stop sign. Is it a sign or a symbol? It is both. The distinction between the two is as follows: A sign generally has only one or few *accepted* meanings which are agreed upon by society or by a group of people, and which stays the same until people agree to change them. A stop sign remains a stop sign until society decides to change its meaning into something else. When we perceive that sign, we automatically think about its accepted meaning. All signs have symbolic meanings, but symbols are not always signs. Therefore, a sign is a particular limitation of a symbol.

The extent of the meaning of a symbol is far greater than that of a sign; it is, in fact, limitless in openings and possibilities.

Table 1: Signs versus Symbols	
SIGN:	SYMBOL:
1. Focused	Diffuse
2. Limited	Limitless
3. One or few meanings	Multiple meanings
4. Easy to change	Difficult to change
5. Conscious	Subconscious

When we perceive a symbol, it triggers emotional responses in the subconscious which summon us to feel everything we ever experienced in connection with that particular symbol – be they situations, facts, judgments, actions, thoughts, feelings, sensations or messages. Seeing a knife subconsciously elicits all our past memories when we cut bread, cooked, carved wood, fought, gardened or played with a knife.

We may choose to pick one or several memories according to our present needs. We may choose to ignore them all and that is fine also. By ignoring or by attuning, we shape different sets of experiences that we are going to share with the world. One set of experiences is not better than another, they are just different (even though we often judge them as better or worse).

Nature's Language

We all have emotional reflexes or reactions toward symbols. Emotions are a fundamental way of communication in the universe. We need to emotionally relate to things in order to understand them. For example, a movie that elicits absolutely no emotional reaction in us (not even boredom) is virtually nonexistent to us. It does not communicate anything of value to us; in fact, we wouldn't even choose to see that movie. It simply would not appear into our lives. Emotional communication is one of the highest form of truth for oneself – it goes beyond words or socially accepted forms of expression.

By evoking emotions, symbols remain in our awareness, where their most important function is to help us relate to the environment in a meaningful way. The heart, for example, is a symbol of love, connection and harmony. Fairy tales are filled with such symbols that bypass the logical mind and access our hearts directly. Symbolically, we can say that the symbols themselves are perceived with the heart. When our heart is receptive and loving, we are receptive to the language of nature. The more our heart is blocked with resistance, doubt or disharmony, the more disturbed our reception of love will be.

Subconscious Communications

Symbols are probably the most powerful means of communication on the subconscious level. They have been termed the currency within the subconscious level. For example, the color gray represents neutrality and noninvolvement. When someone decides to wear gray clothes, this person subconsciously communicates that he or she wishes to remain uninvolved with something. Subconsciously, we all understand this, even though our conscious mind may not be aware of it. The color of our clothes, our facial expressions, our gait and many other such symbols provide subliminal clues about our internal emotional state at any given moment. Most of these messages are subconscious. We may not even know why we picked certain clothes – they simply resonated with our need of the day.

When we look at a face, that face resonates with us in a certain way and we instinctively tune in and know that person's character. Consciously, we may perceive only a small part of the message, most likely the part that society dictates to be appropriate.

However, there is a lot more information being processed on the subconscious level.

Based on this phenomenon, some people have concluded that we use only 10% of our brain. We may indeed use no more than 10% for conscious logical thinking processes, but conscious thinking is only the tip of the iceberg. The other 90% of our mental potential is busy with subconscious processes which are, as yet, only dimly understood by the mainstream scientific community. It appears, however, that these deep subconscious layers are indispensable to the functioning of the superficial conscious 10%. The intricacies, subtleties and power of this subconscious realm are a profound and truthful aspect of ourself. But because of this subtlety and complexity, we are rarely aware of our subconscious messages to the point of being able to influence or change them.

Symbols are Triggers

Subconscious symbolic messages can trigger powerful emotional reactions. We often wonder , in retrospect, why we felt so shocked or revolted at a certain event. These responses, urges or feelings hit us many times without any logical explanation. For example, flashing lights are known to provoke seizures in certain individuals. An event or a symbol is not per se good or bad, but our attachments, needs and judgments are coloring the way we see and process it. A survivor of a plane crash is likely to perceive the symbol of an airplane differently than a pilot of a pleasure airline. It is the passenger himself, not the symbol (the airplane in this case), that attaches positive or negative feelings to airplanes. The degree to which we are affected by different life events depends largely upon the way we subconsciously process these events. I will show you how to tap into this subtle process and use that information in the case of illness.

Symbols Interconnect

Symbols combine with others and merge into new symbols that form a larger whole. By analyzing the symbolic messages or colors, feelings, sensations, etc., we subconsciously receive messages about the whole. For example, when looking at a house we may formulate an idea about the personality and mood of its residents. We can speculate about their culture, tendencies, education, financial status and lifestyle, just by the way they maintain their house.

Everything is a Symbol

Perception means reception of vibration on the same wave length. To attune means to become at one with a source, to vibrate at the same wave length and to experience the same vibrations. Our thought patterns manifest into reality so that the reality will mirror our thoughts. In other words, what is being symbolized to us is nothing other than our own self! We attract people and situations that symbolically mirror our concepts, attitudes and thought patterns. I will go so far as to say that we cannot even perceive anything that we are not attuned to. This means that, in order for us to be aware of an object, the object has to vibrate at the same wave length as we do. This phenomenon is called resonance.

The principle of resonance implies that, when we focus on negative qualities in others, we are focusing on our own corresponding negative emotions. We manifest what we fear. We cannot see the greediness in politicians without resonating with our greediness. We cannot appreciate the courage of explorers without resonating with our personal courage. This principle is valid for individuals, groups, corporations and even nations. The more we resist or criticize something, the more that something will be present. By breaking the cycle of resistance, we can learn to notice our own patterns, love them and change them.

The Power of Thoughts

Our thoughts are the sparks that put the engine of action into motion. Everything in the cosmos begins as a thought form. If we want to go Hawaii, we first have the desire to go, then make our travel arrangements, and then take the trip. A simple thought has the power to move us and make us travel hundreds of miles. All that humanity has ever created – roads, cities, cultures and whole civilizations – was first born as a thought in somebody's mind. Moreover, a vast majority of life's experiences are provoked by thought patterns that arise from the subconscious level.

However, our conscious thoughts *can* influence subconscious thought patterns. Obviously, we first must become aware of them. By becoming aware of a subconscious process, we expand our sphere of influence in life and gain greater clarity to help solve problems on a conscious level. Once redirected, the new conscious thought patterns may then enter the subconscious and shape a new reality around us.

Symbolic Mirroring

The environment serves us by resonating with our thought patterns and by symbolically saying: "Look around, this is what you believe. Do you like it? Then you can keep it! If you don't, you can change it!" It is this simple.

Here are some examples of mirroring at work: When I have an angry person around me, then I look for what might be angering me. If a workaholic shows up in my life, I check how I feel about the workaholic (or perhaps the lazy) side of me. If someone doesn't get along with their children, they might investigate their life issues around their creations, whatever those may be: ideas, philosophies, machineries, plans, a new project, etc. If a complainer is nagging us, it is time to ask about the complaints we might have, but if someone treats us with respect then we can take credit for this as well.

Mirroring is nature's effective way of reflecting back to us some aspect that we were not willing to otherwise examine. Every problem or illness arises to teach us something; our conditions are custom made for our personal needs. The implications are far reaching. They are also extremely positive since they teach that our circumstances exist to help us grow and, in fact, nothing is here to get us. The notions of good and bad then become nothing more than arbitrary labels.

The things that happen in our lives are the things we ask for in some way, usually subconsciously. We need them, whether we like it or not.

Einstein's theory of relativity is not only applicable to the physical world, but to our psychological settings as well. What is good for you might be detrimental for me. When we view life events from a higher spiritual perspective, they all can be seen as opportunities to experience, change and grow. Many ancient masters have taught this: "You are the center of your universe. Change yourself and then everything will change around you."

In order to influence and honor our subconscious needs, we all need to remember the old quote, "Ask and you shall be given." Through careful asking we can start rebuilding our lives step-by-step. Asking and believing are tools of tremendous personal and collective power.

Symbols Shape the Future

Every event from the past or present becomes a new symbol for the future. The so-called unused 90% of our brain processes information in very systematic ways. Every object, color, sound or feeling that we encounter becomes endowed with a specific meaning, ready to be accessed in time of need. Data is being compared, analyzed, classified, synthesized, and then decisions and solutions are offered to the conscious mind. The solutions are created according to our previous subconscious programming from our specific needs of experience.

Symbols and Society

Symbolic messages are processed according to our personal needs, but also according to society's needs. Much of our current cultural focus is on war, intolerance, excessively hard work and competition. Our society believes that life is a struggle, a fight, a battlefield; and values people for being competitive fighters. We fight in life. We fight against the competition. We fight against disease. We may fight against our weight. We fight against just about everything. Why is there so much violence around us? Because we have created an environment that mirrors our beliefs about life. This is by itself not good or bad; it is an innocent reflection of our collective consciousness. Once we understand this and change, fighting will disappear.

The fighting drive is complemented by another factor – that of victimhood. Half of America is on the brink of collapse, exhausted from the mad race of competition and desperately lacking harmony and spirituality in the family. We are locked in the belief that we are victims of society, the government, diseases, and many other imaginary monsters. This belief can be convenient because it seems easier to blame somebody else and do nothing, than to take responsibility and find solutions. By believing in victimhood we just avoid looking deeper for answers within us. It is easier to escape from work and blame a bug, than to openly acknowledge that we need to resolve our anger at our boss. The bug or disease might be an association or even a consequence of our thought patterns and beliefs.

A disease is part of us. We don't need to fight *against* disease. By fighting it we fight against that part of ourselves. Time has come to move beyond disease by *understanding* it at a deeper level. In this way we won't ignore the problem or try to cut it out, but instead we may learn how to openly face it and embrace its implications. Once this understanding has taken place, the urge toward fighting and resistance turns to a desire for compassion and cooperation.

Some say we live in an age that requires us to learn about tolerance, peace, openness and flexibility. We learn these values by evaluating what our surroundings are reflecting back to us. Slowly and gradually some companies and corporations cease to believe that competition is the key to success and are beginning to focus on cooperation instead. By recognizing the mirror of fighting and intolerance, society as a whole may conclude that more tolerance and understanding are needed, and these qualities can thus be brought out.

From this point of view, the collective attachment to the symbol of the "warrior" is gradually shifting to a new "adventurer" type. Our attitudes are slowly changing from "life is a struggle" to "life is an adventure." I believe the trend will gain momentum. More and more people will refuse to believe that they have to work themselves sick, or that everyone is out to get everyone else. They are refusing to believe in victimhood and beginning to recognize that we as individuals, families and groups are not separate from society. They will begin to mirror that we are an integral part of nature and the universe. Most of all, I believe we will see more people taking back their power of creation.

Symbols and Information

It has been my experience that illness is an expression of issues that need to be faced at different levels of our consciousness. Illness points out a lack of communication with a hidden aspect within us. The purpose of this communication is to reintegrate and heal those forgotten parts of ourselves.

When we are engaged in a thought pattern that is not for our highest good, our subconscious sends us warning signals long before a disease appears. It communicates symbolically through feelings, sensations or emotions so that we will make the appropriate changes in our lives. These subtle impulses are telling us what our true self needs in order to ensure our optimal well-being and evolution. If we ignore these *emotions*, there will be *mental* thoughts bugging us about what we should or shouldn't do.

At times, we don't understand such a thought message either and fail to acknowledge it. It might seem easy to blame something external and feel victimized. However, if the subtle emotional and mental messages remain unacknowledged, they eventually manifest more physically, in the form of a *physical* disability or a serious illness. Once they have advanced to the state of illness or pain, they are not so easy to ignore anymore.

Until we understand, consciously or subconsciously, that a disease represents a specific communication from our own self, true healing cannot take place. Disease is a self-referral communication that intends to create healing.

When mechanics was the most advanced scientific accomplishment, we explained everything as being akin to machinery; the whole universe was seen as a big clockwork. Then the focus shifted to electronics, and our brains became likened to computers. Now, the information highway is fashionable; therefore the approach to disease as informational disturbance can become fashionable only now. The symbolic approach to disease is in fact an informational approach, linking messages to events.

The language of nature is universal and symbolic. Information is symbolic. Every illness, every emotion, every symptom or energetic imbalance has a message. It is safe to consider our ailments our allies, because they show us the way to healing and the path to fulfillment.

Symbols and Change

In case of an illness, the easy solution is to be willing, receptive and understanding. The hard way is to get sicker until the message is acknowledged. We may even choose to die without ever acknowledging the message. By becoming more ill, our system is sounding the alarm to tell us that we are straying further from the path our innermost self wants to take. The first step in healing requires the willingness to examine our current issues, and the willingness to change. When we are truly ready to change, our inner self receives the message: "I am willing to change; please show me the way." Our inner, true self is always listening to our messages and always responding, whether we perceive it or not.

At first, we don't even have to know how or what to change; all that is required is the willingness to change and receive guidance. If we believe in change, we will spontaneously manifest it in our lives. When we ask for specific changes, the universe responds according to those specific requests in terms of our belief system. The universe is always allowing and never forcing issues. However, if our belief system is so rigid that we would rather die than change, then the illness goes on. The universe does not force issues, WE do.

It is important to be specific when asking for something. If we are not sure what it is that we want, we send back a message to the universe, "Please put it on hold until I decide." And that is exactly what will happen. For example, someone may look for a perfect mate, but unless they define in detail what a perfect mate means to them, it won't happen. The process of finding the perfect mate is either put on hold until they clarify those details, or they attract someone who is most perfect for recognizing which details are not yet clear to them.

Symbols and Imagination

Nature communicates through symbols. We can also communicate through symbols. When we do this, we operate at the same vibration as nature, which is the most natural and truthful way of expression. A very powerful way to accomplish this communication is to imagine the result we want – the healing we desire, the places we want to visit, the objects we want to acquire. Imagination is one of our most powerful tools for progress, yet it often discarded by our society. We tend to forget that imagination is the most crucial part in all scientific advancements. Without imagination our civilization would stagnate and die.

Half a century ago, Einstein said that imagination is more important than knowledge. This is because imagination carries the powers of manifestation and gives us the ability to overcome our physical limitations. Imagination is our projection into the future or into other dimensions of reality. Once we discard our belief in victimhood, it becomes much easier to change our life circumstances. It is our right, challenge and adventure to create whatever we desire.

To consistently manifest our desires through imagination is an art that one doesn't master overnight. There are many interferences that can amplify, change or block this delicate process. Nevertheless, when we imagine something we truly need, and we trust and believe in the process, we are going to get it.

The only kind of healing is self-healing. Nobody can heal us if we are not willing to change; healers and medications work only if we allow them to. The same principle is true for surgery, alternative healing methods, placebo, or whatever else. This is why generations of medications change with generations of people. For example, what worked wonderfully for headaches fifty years ago is not working anymore. This is because our society, and thus our medical establishment, changed a belief system. If we, as a

---

Table 2:
Functions of a Symbol

---

1. Symbolic mirror
2. Opportunity for symbolic attunement
3. Gateway to the subconscious
4. Nature's messenger
5. Link between various experiences
6. Trigger of emotional reactions
7. Transmitter of information
8. Tool for imagination and intuition
9. Catalyst for change

society or scientific establishment, believe that a drug works, a majority of experiments will confirm that it does.

It all seems as though the universe were playing a game with us. The rule of the game is straightforward: "We are allowed to live life according to our free will." Obviously, there is a never-ending flow of interactions and power plays between individual beliefs and society's beliefs. Sometimes they are contradictory, but the overall result of this interaction will mirror our overall belief system. Even the contradictions are part of our belief system and shape the society the way it is. Our experiments will confirm our beliefs in a majority of cases. The consequences are mind boggling: When we change our beliefs, society, medicine and everything will change.

Presently, the scientific understanding of the process of disease is very limited. We don't know the underlying cause of diseases. Scientifically, the blaming finger has been pointed at enzymes, cholesterol, wrong diet or lack of exercise. Through this kind of blame, we merely exchange one mystery for another of a different nature. We hide behind definitions and technical words, but the issue is far from solved.

Some say there are no incurable diseases, only incurable individuals. This would imply that YOU are the best doctor in the world, even though you may not know it. When you go to the doctor, you, in fact, give a part of your healing powers to him and his drugs (there is nothing wrong in that) because you believe in them. They work for you according to your beliefs and education. In our culture, we were educated to trust more in the healing powers of others than in our own. We can choose to change that. Because of our education, we recognize that doctors and healers are fulfilling a valuable function for us. Very few people are willing and trained to take responsibility into their own hands. It just seems much easier to take a pill and believe everything will be all right, than to face issues and take responsibility for the whole healing process.

Time has come for many to take a deeper look at their ability to heal. Many are already seeing beyond the surface of societal beliefs and finding a whole new world. They empower themselves and live a life that they choose and believe in. The more people choose to do this, the more society will change.

Part II

THE FIVE ELEMENTS

❖ ❖ ❖

"Therefore I speak to them in parables;
because they seeing, see not; and hearing,
they hear not; neither do they understand."

❖ ❖ ❖

NETWORKS

Traditional Chinese medicine has existed for thousands of years and survived the trial of time. What we now call science did not exist in those days. I personally believe that no ineffective healing method can survive more than a century at the most. This is why I chose to investigate Chinese philosophy. I found many fascinating concepts worthy of study; among them a select, well-rounded system of symbols that is based on a long, unbroken tradition of successful healing practice.

Traditional Chinese philosophy divides the energetic flow within the human body into five organ-networks which correspond to five phases. The physiology of the entire body, as well as the physiology of nature, is described in terms of the relationship between these phases. Organ networks operate in pairs; when one network is disturbed it affects the other in specific ways. Each network is composed of a solid organ in pair with a hollow organ (as defined by the ancients). All networks also have specific associated emotions, thought patterns, glands, joints and other body parts that operate in close connection with one another and are symbolically interrelated. Together, they give an understanding of the way the universe functions in terms of different aspects or phases. Together, the symbolically interconnected aspects of a network (such as purification, spring, green, etc.) form a phase, just as spring is one seasonal phase and summer is another.

The networks are also symbolically associated with specific seasons, sounds, directions, actions and all cycles and aspects of nature. By understanding these connections, we may learn how to energetically amplify or purify the networks through certain symbolic activities. For a better understanding of the above concepts please refer to **Chart 1**.

However, even in this profoundly insightful system of knowledge, the underlying cause of illness has become lost in the vast complexity of symbols. The Chinese tradition holds that we are the victims of outside forces (wind, cold, dampness, dryness, etc.).

It also needs to be made clear that not all ideas in this book are derived from traditional Chinese medicine. The Chinese system is utilized only in **Part II**, and only because it offers a systematic approach to qualities that might otherwise seem unrelated.

Despite these drawbacks, traditional Chinese medicine has a lot of symbolic potential which we will explore by studying the networks one by one. In order to better understand how these chapters are structured, it is useful to look at **Chart 1** for a general overview and reference. All of the physical structures and corresponding symbols are discussed in terms of phases, which is why they are discussed together. It may be useful to have the chart in front of you for the whole length of this chapter. For a schematic and brief understanding of organ functions, see **Figure 1**.

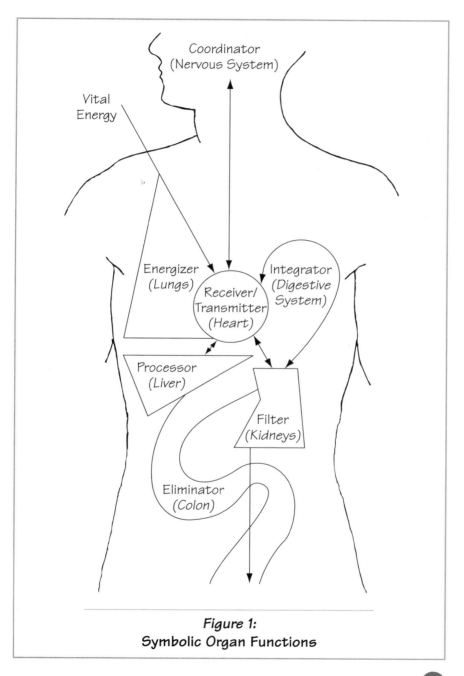

Figure 1:
Symbolic Organ Functions

Chart 1:
Five Phase Correspondences

	I:	II:	III:	IV:	V:
Function	Purification	Circulation	Digestion	Respiration	Elimination
Organ/solid	Liver	Heart	Spleen/pancreas	Lungs	Kidneys
Organ/hollow	Gallbladder	Small intestine	Stomach	Large intestine	Bladder
Color	Green	Red	Yellow (orange)	White	Gray, deep blue, brown, black
Flavor	Sour	Bitter	Sweet	Hot, pungent	Salty
Emotion	Anger	Joy	Sympathy	Grief	Fear
Sound	Shouting	Laughter	Singing	Weeping	Groaning
Direction	Up	Outward	Horizontal	Down	Inward
Sense	Sight	Touch/speech	Taste	Smell	Hearing
Head part	Eyes	Tongue	Mouth	Nose	Ears
Secretion	Tears	Sweat	Saliva	Nasal fluid	Urine
Season	Spring	Summer	Indian summer	Autumn	Winter
Climate	Wind	Heat	Dampness	Dryness	Cold
Injurious entrance	Back of neck	Mouth	Feet	Nose	Shins

(Chart 1 continued)

Head system	Planning, decision-making	Commanding to Action	Imagining	Establishing Rhythmic Order	Persevering by will power
Tonifying activity	Reading	Walking	Sitting	Lying	Standing
Body part	Muscles/sinews (action)	Vascular system	Flesh/muscles (tone)	Skin	Bones/marrow, teeth
Body action	Wrenching, pulling	Joyless, blazing	Retching, moistening	Coughing	Trembling, quivering
Associated body part	Nails	Complexion	Lips	Body hair	Head hair
Glands	Gonads	Pituitary	Thymus	Thyroid	Adrenal
Body smell	Rancid	Scorched	Fragrant	Rotten	Putrid
Joints	Shoulders	Elbows	Hips	Wrists	Knees, ankles
Major vitamins	A, B_2	B_3, B_5, C	B_1, B_6	E	D
Minerals	Copper, iron	Potassium, sodium	Manganese, zinc	Phosphorous	Magnesium, calcium
Organ/solid: full	1 to 3 am	11 am to 1 pm	9 to 11 am	3 to 5 am	5 to 7 pm
Organ/hollow: full	11 pm to 1 am	1 to 3 pm	7 to 9 am	5 to 7 am	3 to 5 pm

THE PURIFICATION NETWORK: LIVER/GALLBLADDER

The liver is the hardest working organ of the body and is involved in all of the metabolic pathways. It regulates the metabolism of proteins, fats and sugars and coordinates coagulation and blood pressure. The liver is essential in balancing water and electrolytes, and participates in the synthesis and activities of hormones and enzymes. Moreover, the liver is involved in lymph production and circulation, vitamin and micro-element balance in the body; it participates in heat production and is the major detoxifier of the body.

Nutrients, once absorbed, are brought to the liver where they are processed or detoxified and then released into the circulation to be used by the whole body. The liver's secretory product is named bile; it is stored in the gallbladder underneath the liver. From the gallbladder, bile is released into the digestive tract by a process synchronized with meals and other natural cycles. Bile aids in the absorption of fats and Vitamins A, D, E and K, through the intestinal wall. Toxins are thus modified, processed and transformed in the liver, making it the major organ of purification, detoxification and metabolic regulation in the body. The

---

Table 3:
Liver Functions

1. Metabolism of proteins, fats and sugars
2. Coagulation and regulation of blood pressure
3. Balancing of water and electrolytes
4. Synthesis and regulation of hormones and enzymes
5. Lymph and bile production
6. Balancing of vitamins and micro-elements
7. Energy and heat regulation
8. Storage of nutrients
9. Purification and elimination of toxins

---

gallbladder then stores and regulates the discharge products of the liver.

Symbolically, the liver purifies our toxic situations and problems that are not in line with our plans and visions. By releasing bile at the most appropriate time, the gallbladder makes decisions involving the present and the future. Ailments of the liver or gallbladder may symbolically indicate anger and hostility or a refusal to process life and live the way one would like to. For a better understanding of the liver's position in the body and its relationship with other organs, please see **Figure 2**.

Symbolic Function

The liver symbolically relates to everything that suggests action, movement, building or processing, which is associated with the spring season – a universal symbol for new actions, new beginnings, planning and building. Wind is also related to this network as a symbol of action and perpetual movement. Purification is an act of balancing. The associated color is green, the balancing color in the center of the solar spectrum.

Emotions

Feelings manifest at different levels of intensity. Frustration, for example, can develop into anger and then rage. When feelings are suppressed, the corresponding emotional reaction is frustration. When they are partially expressed, the reaction becomes anger. When they are acted and shouted out, people call it rage. Symbolically, we can say that anger is a response to a situation that did not come out as we planned. Our expectations are not met, we experience this as instability, and the situation has to be processed again. Symbolically this processing is accomplished by the liver, which may become overworked. Anger is, in fact, a refusal to see life in a new, unexpected way. Next time you find yourself angry, I suggest you give your liver a break and look around for an unexpected outcome of a situation.

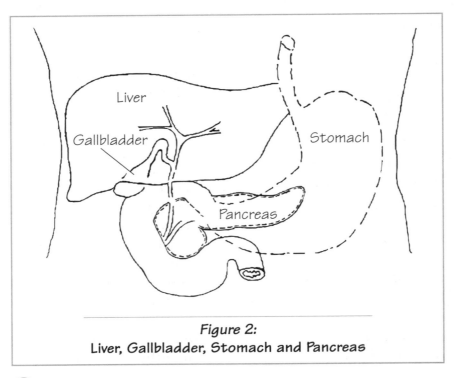

Figure 2:
Liver, Gallbladder, Stomach and Pancreas

Senses

There is a well-known symbolic correlation between liver and eyesight. When the liver becomes toxic and overworked, vision will weaken. In scientific terms, there is no apparent explanation. In symbolic terms, however, when our plans are not turning out as we had expected, we subconsciously refuse to see and accept this. These subliminal messages we send to ourself will eventually add up. The mind gets the message and acts accordingly. In extreme situations, somebody may be blinded by rage.

Organs

Muscles and sinews (small fluid sacks that ease movements) are associated with the liver in their capacity to move, accomplish action and produce change.

Glands

Building blocks for sexual hormones are manufactured in the liver. When the liver becomes clogged and does not function well, sexual hormone production is disturbed and the sexual drive decreases.

Vitamins and Minerals

Vitamins A and B_2 are stored in the liver and have a role in the metabolic processing of proteins, fats and sugars. They also improve eyesight and protect the liver from toxins. Sexual organs, skin and hair need Vitamins A and B_2 in order to thrive. Copper and iron are important for healthy liver activity. They play a role in the production and storage of energy, cellular respiration and protection from oxidants, but are also catalysts in oxidative processes. When the metabolism of copper and iron is disrupted, two different diseases (Wilson's disease and hemochromatosis) may occur, which are characterized mainly by overloaded stores of copper or iron in the liver.

Timing

According to Chinese traditional philosophy, there are energetic pathways within the body which are activated in a strict sequence during a 24-hour cycle. Each organ has two hours of maximum energetic activity in each day. Symbolically at 11:00 pm, while we sleep, the gallbladder works at maximum rate to process what the liver has accumulated during that day. Its activity further stimulates liver activity which takes place over two hours later. All these processes happen while we are resting and dream activity is low, so our activities don't interfere. Like a big food store, the liver cleanses and puts everything in order during the night, when the flow of customers is minimal.

THE CIRCULATION NETWORK: HEART/SMALL INTESTINE

This network represents the fire element, heat, summer and the color red. We can compare the heart to a pump that distributes blood throughout the body at a specific rate. The rate of the heart is the rate of the life we have.

Symbolic Function

Symbolically the heart receives and redistributes emotions, love, vitality and strength. It is a symbolic receiver and transmitter. By redistributing emotions, the heart maintains the connection between the inner life and the external world. The continuous pumping of blood to all the cells is nourishing and life sustaining; it also supports communication among them. From the quality and quantity of blood passing through, a cell receives information about each organ's functional status. For example, a muscle cell is aware (through the quality of blood) of how well the liver is processing, how much the lungs are oxygenating and how well the kidneys are filtering, etc.

The qualities of heat and joy are always expanding and radiating outward. Obviously, summer is the season associated with heat, expansion, joy and exuberance. Skin complexion is a good indicator of the status of our vascular function, as it varies according to circumstances. During regular activity it appears pale pink; faster circulation or congestion turns it reddish; while slower circulation makes the complexion appear blue. An area of congestion (lots of stagnating blood) is symbolic of an emotional hangup or stagnation toward the symbolic meaning of that body part. All inflammatory diseases show this major symptom and can be approached from this perspective.

Normal circulation gives an appealing aromatic smell to the body. The characteristic smell of disturbed or restricted circulatory function is scorched or burnt. I encounter it often in the hospital around dying people and those with vascular diseases. Bitter, the flavor associated with this network, stimulates the salivary and gastric secretions and helps assimilation. (This is probably why appetizers and digestive aids are often bitter.)

Emotions

The heart symbolically assimilates emotional signals and transmits them to every cell of the body. It is the function of the heart to receive and spread love, joy and fulfillment. As the heart (ful)fills the vessels with blood, it symbolically fulfills our life with love and joy. Symbolically the heart provides communication, support, warmth and energy for the creation and growth of every new cell, both physically and spiritually.

Heart

The heart absorbs emotions, spreads joy and maintains peace. Our blood symbolically represents the love, joy and nourishment of life itself as it flows through the body, bringing vitality to the cells, tissues and organs. Blood disturbances and diseases of the blood, such as leukemia, may represent a disturbance of the love, joy and nourishment flowing through us, or it may signify some internal reaction to joy and nourishment.

Cardiovascular problems are a fashionable subject because heart attack is one of the leading causes of death these days. I find few heart attack patients who are noticeably radiant and joyful or vibrant with inner harmony and unconditional love for everything and everybody. Rather, they tend to be competition oriented and are trained to distrust, oppose and fight people. This is just a consequence of an educational system. Love and cooperation are not the main focus in most people's daily routine. To some extent, we all display some of these characteristics. Heart attack patients are, in fact, trapped in strict, rigid lives, and so are their arteries – strict and rigid. Their lesson is about flexibility and love.

During a heart attack, a person experiences pain on the front side of the chest. This symptom symbolically translates into a denial of our ability to give unconditional love. The inability to love someone mirrors in fact an inability to love those aspects of oneself, which are symbolically represented by another person. Some people would rather die than love themselves. These denials are very specifically oriented toward something or someone in their life.

Heart attacks are physically manifested by clogs that block the blood flow in a heart artery. The location of the blockage also has a specific significance (e.g., right, left, front or bottom of the heart – see the index at the end of the book). Clogs become lodged in places that contain heavy fatty deposits, where we symbolically feel the need to protect ourselves and resist the flow of life. Without love and joy, life might (symbolically) not seem worth living, and this is exactly what is being manifested in a heart attack.

Think about these concepts for a while, then look around you and within yourself. It is very challenging to be uncompromisingly honest with oneself, but it always pays off. Are you immersed in struggle and competition? Then sooner or later you will manifest experiences that confirm those beliefs. If there is generosity and trust flowing in your heart, then those are the qualities that will shape your future. The choice really is yours!

Small Intestine

The small intestine is doing the same job as the heart, but on a different level. While the heart assimilates the emotional world, the small intestine assimilates the physical world into the body. Food is absorbed by the intestines according to our needs for nourishment. After absorption, the food particles enter the portal vein (the vessel that connects the intestine with the liver). All nutrients except fats travel from the small bowel directly to the liver where they are purified and then sent out to the heart for distribution to each cell of the body. The majority of fats, however, are not routed to the liver for processing. The symbolic explanation for this is simple: Fats are symbolic of protection.

All cell and nuclear membranes consist of fats, whose role is to protect the cells from outside injuries and imbalances while maintaining the internal patterns and individuality of the cells. Fatty tissues function as heat and electric insulators, which are symbolically translated into emotional and mental insulators. When we feel threatened, protection becomes top priority. We put our usual activity on hold and take care of safety matters first. This is the symbolic reason why fats are not required to undergo preliminary processing in the liver before assuming their role as protectors. From the small intestine, fats pass through the lymphatic circulatory system and are quickly delivered into the blood stream, being distributed to the tissues first and only later to the liver for ulterior processing.

Senses

There is general agreement that red is the color of fire, symbolizing energy, force, passion, activity and strength. The corresponding emotion of the fire element is joy, which is transported by the blood to every cell. Blood also carries in a liquid (emotional) form many life components, including oxygen – the symbolic spiritual spark of life.

Vitamins and Minerals

It is well known that Vitamins C, B_3 and B_5 are important for the circulatory system. The strengthening and tonifying effect of Vitamin C on capillaries is well documented. Vitamin B_3, or Niacin, stimulates the circulation and may even produce hot flashes when ingested. Vitamin B_5, or pantothenic acid, plays a vital role in the synthesis of hemoglobin (an important element that gives the blood its red appearance and carries oxygen to the tissues). Sodium and potassium have a positive effect in maintaining a good blood volume balance. Sodium and potassium will be further analyzed later in the book when we explain symbolic cell function.

Timing

Noon is the time of day when the effects of heat and activity are at their peak. The energy of the heart is full between 11:00 am and 1:00 pm, followed by the small intestine which peaks between 1:00 and 3:00 pm. This is why most cultures eat their largest meal of the day at shortly past noon when the digestive energy is utilized most efficiently. This is being changed in western countries, but the benefits of such a trend are questionable, as our biological clocks are set to function in harmony with universal principles, rather than business calendars.

THE DIGESTION NETWORK:
SPLEEN/PANCREAS/STOMACH

Chemical digestion of food begins in the stomach. Later, in the small intestines, pancreatic juices (which contain the most powerful digestive enzymes) break down the food elements into fats, sugars and proteins. A special secretion of the pancreas helps the body to assimilate and digest sugars.

The function of the spleen is to digest old or worn out red blood cells and other elements of blood that are no longer necessary, such as microbes and foreign substances. After filtering the blood, the spleen acts like a sponge that absorbs and stores blood in pools to be sent out into the circulation when the body requires it. In this way, the spleen controls the circulating blood volume. The spleen also produces antibodies which help our body destroy foreign substances that cannot be digested in a normal way. If necessary, the spleen can also activate white blood cells to digest potentially harmful substances and microorganisms. In summary, this network regulates and distributes unprocessed materials of food and emotions in order to fuel the body, mind and feelings.

Symbolic Function

People with good digestion are symbolically well prepared to digest life. Those who do not assimilate life experiences very well, may fall into the habit of eating a lot, as eating is a symbolic substitute for assimilating life events. We tend to overeat when bored, but forget to eat when we are really engrossed in an experience.

The color yellow is associated with this network, symbolizing cheerfulness and easy assimilation. Yellow stands for relaxation and dilatation, which is exactly what our digestive organs do when we sit down to eat. Relaxation also implies relief from burdens or restrictions; therefore eating is sometimes used as an escape from stressful realities.

We all long to experience and digest the sweetness, love and harmony of life. A special substance called insulin, secreted by the pancreas, helps the sugar within our food become absorbed by the cells via the cell membranes. When we experience a disturbance about accepting our sweet feelings, we can manifest a condition that lets sweetness pass right through the body without being absorbed into the cells. This disease is called *diabetes mellitus*, which literally means "sugar passes through."

Senses

Taste, on the psychological level, can be considered a selective, predigestive process. Our favorite food tastes good when we are hungry, but neutral right after we eat a plate full of it. Ideally, when our digestive system is balanced, we can rely on taste to tell us what is needed by the body at any given moment. Through the stomach, spleen and pancreas network, we then assimilate and balance the building blocks of life.

However, taste can also indicate emotional imbalances. You may notice that you crave sweets when you need love and affection, while at other times you don't even notice the candies placed just in front of you.

Emotions

The psychological equivalent of welcoming, embracing and absorbing new concepts is called imagination. Through imagination we digest new opportunities, accept new experiences and find new solutions. Imagination is absolutely essential to the well being of people. It is proven that without the creative anticipation of visions, hopes and dreams, we stop growing and die, just as the body dies without food.

On the other hand, when we encounter ideas or experiences that are difficult to face, we may find ourselves mentally rehashing them over and over. This psychological rumination is known as worry. Symbolically, this kind of refusal manifests as retching, clearing the throat, belching, nausea and vomiting, all of which are associated with rejecting or backward movements of the digestive system. By throwing up we symbolically reject an experience. Nausea is one of the most common symptoms in the medical field, as it symbolizes one of the first symptoms of not accepting change.

Vitamins and Minerals

Vitamins B_1 and B_6 are known for their effect in reducing motion sickness (nausea) and improving digestion. Vitamin B_1 maintains balance in the nervous system which is necessary for us to think clearly and be capable of imagination. Vitamin B_1 also helps the forward movement of the digestive system and the absorption of sugars and oxygen into the cells. Vitamin B_6 may relieve the hardening of the arteries, known as arterial sclerosis, which occurs when one's experiences are no longer properly assimilated and the flow of joy in life is restricted (less blood in the arteries).

Manganese and zinc are essential elements that help the body grow by participating in hundreds of chemical reactions that take place inside of us. Many energetic systems and glands in the body utilize manganese to help the fixations of minerals, calcium, iron and vitamins. Its actions strongly correlate with the B vitamin complex and is essential in the proper functioning of the pancreas and in many other energetic processes.

Gland Regulators

The thymus and the spleen are two major regulators of our immune response and work in close connection with the lymphatic system. The way our immune system responds to events is proportional to our enthusiasm for life, our readiness to absorb new experiences, and our openness to an evolutionary path. Fear of vulnerability and the belief that something is out to get us contribute to low immunity.

The body may further develop antibodies against itself. When we are convinced that something is out there to attack us, we develop an internal mirror by creating something inside to attack us. This is known as immunologic disease. All immuno-logic diseases have in common the fact that the body attacks its own structures. Symbolically this translates into a feeling of not accepting who we are, not acknowledging ourselves as creators of our own experiences and acting out the role of a victim. In fact, we then become victims of ourselves, which is exactly what immunologic diseases are about.

Timing

The digestive network energy has its height in the morning hours. Between 7:00 and 9:00 am we begin a new day, ready to absorb new experiences. The energy of the stomach is maximal at this time, followed by the spleen and pancreas energies two hours later. This ensures optimum accumulation and integration of new experiences into the whole.

THE RESPIRATION NETWORK:
LUNGS AND LARGE INTESTINE

Through the lungs we take in the vital breath of life. We also receive spiritual energy and guidance. This is so important that we cannot live without it, even for five minutes. Respiration sets up the cycles of life through inhalation and exhalation, which instills rhythm and order in the body, mind and emotions.

Symbolic Function

Respiration symbolically defines the extent to which we can expand (accept) and contract (reject) life. The lungs, the only internal organ with direct access to the exterior of the body, sets boundaries between the internal and external world. Through the lungs we delineate an inner border or meeting place between us and the universe. The skin plays a similar role by defining our external border or contact surface with the environment. Lungs and skin are reshaped and restructured according to conditions and needs. When there is no involvement in an activity, for example, the breath is shallow. A significant part of the blood that flows to the lungs is then shunted (in other words, it does not fully reach the lungs). This means that the connection between blood and air, between inner and outer, is minimal. When we become involved in an enjoyable activity, our breath deepens. More blood vessels take on more oxygen and the energy flow through the body is increased. The symbolic purpose of inhalation is to create new open spaces for life experiences, ideas and emotions. Old patterns, feelings and emotions are eliminated through exhalation.

Every breath is a symbolic step forward in life. The role of the lungs and large intestines is to take in what we need and discard what has become obsolete. The old and useless is being expelled by lungs and large intestines, given back to nature and recycled. Laughing, singing, crying all have the power to release a great deal of pressure by enhancing our respiration. Old fears and resentments may be released simply through deep breathing. It comes as no surprise that deep breathing is a technique used since ancient times to promote well-being and longevity.

The breath rate influences all other processes in our lives. There are important proportional correlations between breathing and other physiological processes, the most well known of them being the heart beat/respiration ratio of four-to-one (4:1). When this proportion becomes disturbed, our physical integrity is at risk.

The lungs symbolize life itself. White, the associated color, stands for purity, complexity and spiritual balance of life. Whenever we disregard our hidden need for balance or resist life experiences exactly the way they are, then grief and sorrow are bound to follow. Symbolically, everything then seems to be falling, contracting, rotting in the air and large intestines.

Organs

Lungs symbolically represent the ability to take in, welcome, receive and let go. They are the most spiritual organ of the body, symbolizing allowance, connection, receptivity, processing and elimination all in one. Just as sunlight is a synthesis of all the colors, so the activity of the lungs can be regarded as a synthesis of all the major body functions. (**Figure 3** shows the relative position of body organs.)

Emotions

Our lungs help us process grief and sadness. We are all familiar with the tendency to hold our breath when sad or tense. This happens because breathing represents acceptance and letting go – the opposite of holding back. In a medical emergency, one of the first steps in resuscitation is to give the patient oxygen. By breathing deeply, we convey a message to nature (and to the body) that we are now ready to relax, let go of worries and trust in spiritual guidance. Deep breathing can be used as a powerful tool for breaking through any kind of crisis, be it medical, emotional or mental. By inhaling, we accept life to flow in the way it is.

Coughing symbolizes rejection and opposition. We refute what someone says, what we feel or think. Here is a revealing experiment you can do: Next time you cough, recall exactly what you just thought, felt, or heard at that time, and discover the source of your defensive reaction. What is it that your subconscious refuses to accept?

Senses

The sense of smell is associated with breathing; we couldn't smell anything without taking a breath. When our nose is stuffed, we feel stuck in a situation and refuse to flow with it. This is a symbolic rejection of our higher guidance mechanism. During this time, we may ask ourselves questions like "Why always me?" or "Why do I always have to do these things I don't like doing?"

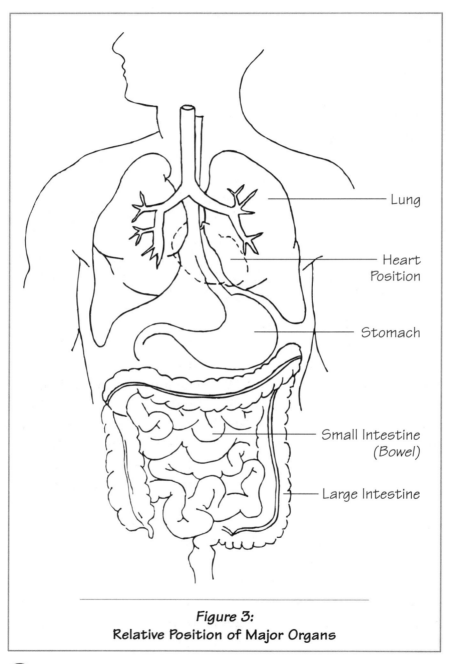

Figure 3:
Relative Position of Major Organs

The answer is always simple, yet difficult to acknowledge: We ourselves have designed life to be exactly the way it is, very carefully, through subconscious choices. People often say of a tragedy, "It could have happened to me." No, it could not and did not, because all life events are carefully planned by the subconscious and they happen for a reason well known by our inner self.

Gland

The thyroid is an endocrine gland located on the lower front side of the neck. It is involved in establishing rhythm and order by setting up cycles and patterns for all the bodily functions. This gland regulates the metabolism (the internal fire) and, similarly to the lungs, gives strength and energy to all the tissues while maintaining the most efficient rhythm for every cell.

Vitamins and Minerals

Vitamin E supports the respiration system. It helps the chemical reaction of life (redox) and promotes the absorption of oxygen at the cellular level. What the lungs accomplish at the macroscopic level (the level of the whole body), Vitamin E repeats at the microscopic, cellular level, by helping the cells to absorb life and adapt as necessary. It protects the cells from toxins by promoting deep breathing at the cellular level (literally and spiritually). Only by accepting life and remaining open to change, can the cells be healthy and function harmoniously. Vitamin E has a strong anti-oxidant effect and is utilized for maintaining the tissues young.

Phosphorus is present in nearly all of the energetic and structural systems of the body (DNA, RNA and phospholipids) and plays a crucial role as an energy source for breathing. Phosphorus is involved in energetic processes that involve energy storing substances like ATP, ADP and others.

Timing

Optimum energy flow in the lungs occurs between 3:00 and 5:00 am. This reflects the notion that we receive much spiritual guidance in our sleep and dreams. Lung activity is helped by the fact that the body is lying down fully relaxed, while the mental barriers and inhibitions are removed. Just before the beginning of a new day, between 5:00 and 7:00 am, the large intestine reaches its zenith of energy by processing and letting go of the past. It is creating open spaces for new ideas, experiences and emotions, and welcomes the new day that is about to dawn.

THE ELIMINATION NETWORK: KIDNEYS AND BLADDER

Elimination is performed through four main organs of the body: kidneys, lungs, large intestine and skin. The kidneys are the most representative elimination organ and are responsible for concentrating, filtering and balancing the body fluids. Kidneys filter salt out of the fluids and eliminate old water (symbolizing emotions), thus maintaining the health of the internal fluids that surround every cell. When the kidneys don't function properly, there is an accumulation of waste products around the cells. Cells then become toxic and deprived of energy, information and vital power.

The kidneys and bladder are located deep in the abdomen (see **Figure 4**). Kidney function is continuous, but the liquid filtered by the kidneys is stored in the bladder and released from time to time. The kidney gets rid of unusable salted substances and excess water amounts (symbolic of emotions). A minimum amount of liquid has to pass through the kidneys in order to dissolve and flush out the toxins; this is why it is important for us to drink water.

Symbolic Functions

Water, the element of life, is flowing and adaptable, as are emotions. Without emotions and feelings, there is no life. Just as we regulate our body fluids mostly on a subconscious level, we also process emotions without being aware of the whole procedure. In the event of a hemorrhage or a swollen, fluid-filled body part, these events call for attention to emotional processes that need to be addressed by the conscious mind.

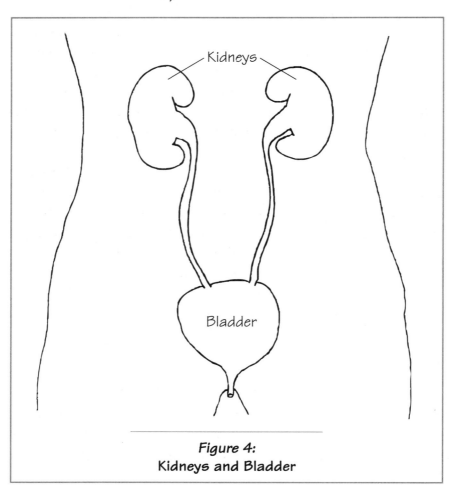

Figure 4:
Kidneys and Bladder

Water is a carrier for dissolved substances. Symbolically, water represents the flow of life that is passing through us. From this life flow we select those experiences and relationships that we need. We also select our obstacles, as well as our joys. Kidney function symbolically represents the ability to flow with life and allow life to flow through us, all the while filtering out and letting go of that which is unnecessary.

The bladder stores and discharges liquid. This symbolically represents our ability to contain and release, in accord with the circumstances. Our emotions are continuously flowing, as is the "water flow" through our kidneys. Throughout the day we experience different groups of emotions like joy or anger, which need to be released several times a day. These releases are symbolized by the bladder releases. By doing this, we symbolically let go of subconscious emotions in order to provide space for new ones.

Ailments of the bladder are about control issues and holding onto old concepts and emotions that need to be eliminated. Water is the symbol for emotions that need to be expressed. It exemplifies a subconscious need to let go and flow with life.

The symbolic colors of the elimination network are dark, such as gray and black. They symbolize underground transformation of new facts, ideas, emotions and circumstances. Black symbolizes detachment and noninvolvement. The black attire of someone in mourning tells us that they are contracting and protecting themselves from disturbing external energies. After some time, they finish the cycle of a hidden regeneration, accept the facts, flow with life and begin a new cycle. (It is interesting to note that certain cultures associate other colors with death and mourning, such as white, representing purity and oneness with the universe, or purple, the color of spirituality – this tells us about their views of death.)

Symbolically, winter has the same significance as the elimination network. Winter is a time of rest and transition. It may seem sad and dreary, if we wish to see it that way, or we can honor it as a necessary part of a new life cycle. Winter represents elimination of the old in order to make room for the new.

Cold causes contraction of matter. During winter, creatures tend to go inward and curl up in their dwellings or underground. Our muscles contract in times of fear, tension and cold. This limits the blood flow, the joy and the power of life. Winter is a time to be on a quiet, regenerative inward stroke that prepares for a new flowering of spring.

Senses

The ears have been correlated with kidneys since ancient times. Kidneys and ears have the same embryological type of tissue at their origin. Medication that damages the kidneys has a hard impact on the hearing sense as well. Patients in renal failure (with blocked kidneys) usually show a corresponding hearing loss. Ears and kidneys have similar shapes and a similar symbolic function – to filter waves (liquids and sounds) in and out of the body.

Emotions

When we find ourselves swimming upstream against the current of life, not understanding why things seem so difficult, the emerging emotion is fear. Fear manifests with control issues and lack of trust in the wisdom that underlies the design of all experiences. The result is contraction, isolation, limitation, and a blocked flow of life.

Salt attracts water in the circulatory system, and the water flushes the kidneys. Therefore, salt helps us deal with internal subconscious emotions. When people crave salt, they are subconsciously processing their fears in order to reestablish the natural flow of life. Salt is serving these people in the process of releasing their fears.

Organs

Shins, knees and ankles initiate the movements of stepping forward, away from the past. When walking, the feet alternate from being the most backward to the most forward parts of the body. Knees and ankles represent the ability to bend, be flexible and support ourselves.

Vitamins and Minerals

Vitamin D is activated by the kidneys and plays a role in the absorption of calcium and phosphorus into the body. Vitamin D also helps with the assimilation of minerals into the bones and kidneys. Magnesium is essential in the energetic metabolism, particularly for bones, and prepares the body to respond to Vitamin D. The balance between calcium and magnesium is indispensable for our well being. A disturbance of this balance causes body quivers, contractions, spasticity, fears and anxiety, as well as heart, kidney and bone problems.

Sometimes kidney stones appear in the body. These hardenings could be considered symbolically equivalent to a new support structure, like a small bone formation out of its normal place. Fear is the underlying issue, which manifests as an attempt to create a fake support system around fearful circumstances.

Timing

Between 3:00 and 5:00 pm, the bladder reaches its energetic climax, allowing us to accumulate, to contain and hold the day's emotions and experiences. Appropriately, the kidney energy peaks next between 5:00 and 7:00 pm, when we contract, filter and let go of the old day in anticipation of a new one.

Part III

THE SYMBOLIC APPROACH TO DISEASE

❖ ❖ ❖

"You must embrace in order to change."

❖ ❖ ❖

SYMBOLIC DISEASE

Perceiving the human being as a whole is a worthwhile goal. It is not always easy to consider every aspect of a human being, much less the myriad interconnections that are at work. However, the more we shift our frame of reference toward a comprehensive vision of human nature and disease, the more we expand our consciousness to new horizons of understandings, possibilities and solutions. Let me demonstrate this in a concrete and practical way.

Science deals with reality by using descriptions or models based on the standards of our current understanding of the physical world. For example, people like to say that the brain is like a computer. This statement recognizes only the computer-like features of the brain; the rest is ignored. The brain may in fact be infinitely superior to a computer, but since the computer is the highest technology we know today, this description is highly valued by us. Obviously, such descriptive models only measure what is mirroring us at a given point in time, whereas the totality is never accessed. Our concepts are limited by our worldly experience and vice versa. This vicious circle greatly affects our level of comprehension and truth.

Lately, the vicious circle has become more and more apparent in science – and is continually baffling everybody. We all know that quantum physics, for example, has established that solid matter is an illusion and that we are all made of vibration. What is less well known are the consequences of this discovery; they are far reaching and absolutely mind blowing. If everyone is vibration, then everyone generates quantum vibrational fields which create multidimensional connections reaching far beyond space and time as we know it. This literally means that our vibrations instantly affect every point in the universe. And, as if this wasn't enough of a mouthful, these quantum fields are actually affecting the past and the future! The religious or philosophical claims of universal oneness have now been stumbled upon by science.

The discoveries of the theory of relativity are no less outrageous. Consider, for example, that you are looking at a beam of light. From your frame of reference, you would say that the light particles are traveling through space. However, from the perspective of the light beam, the beam requires zero time to travel – it travels at infinite speed and reaches every point in the universe simultaneously. Neither space nor time exist for the light ray, so in fact it doesn't travel at all. Time only exists for an outside observer. What's more, the apparent distinction between the observer and the light also ceases to exist. So, from the perspective of the light beam, YOU are the radiating light! Everything becomes one. In a very real way, light is the gateway toward universal oneness. It is hardly coincidental that religions and spiritual teachings abound with the sayings, "God is Light," "God is Love," and "we ARE oneness."

Let's not forget that all of the atoms forming our physical body are nothing but electromagnetic vibrations, so the body is literally made of light. Thoughts and emotions are the results of certain substances and neural connections in the body; these are arranged according to specific atomic and molecular patterns that radiate specific electromagnetic energies. Simply put, our thoughts and emotions, too, consist of nothing but light. And we now know that every light particle and combination of particles that make up who we are (our body, thoughts and emotions) is instantly connected to the entire universe. The theory of relativity implies that there is an underlying unity at the basis of the universe and all of creation. This discovery further indicates that we truly have the power to actually alter any reality and change the universe. Modern quantum physics emphasizes the fact that, in the absence of an observer, the external world does not exist in a well defined sense. The world begins and ends only because of us and only with us. We truly are the center of our universe – any universe we may choose!

There is much more to these fascinating theories of our most advanced scientific minds; you can check them in every book about quantum physics or the theory of relativity. In my next book, I will further explore the scientific connection with the symbolic aspect of reality. For now, let's see if there is a way to capture quantum reality when dealing with disease.

Speech, our mechanism of expression, is a vehicle of emotional communication. We need to take a position relative to an event in order to observe it and talk about it. When an event is subconsciously perceived as neutral, it doesn't resonate with us, so we don't discuss or even notice it. In other words, the world takes its definite shape only in relation to an observer – *you* – as quantum physics would corroborate; so you *are* the creator of your universe.

So, how do we go about creating something good for ourselves?

The answer is: By paying attention. Since we *are* the universe, everything around us is a reflection of the status of our universe. Everything that we may find ourselves talking about is a symbolic mirror of us. All it takes is to watch and listen. We are always expressing to ourselves what's going on – be it "how nice," "how ugly," "how boring" or even "how neutral." That emotional response indicates a deviation from our position of neutrality which makes us pay attention to things. Something can stir us *only* if we have an issue of interest, or a lesson to learn about that issue. This is why, for example, cardiologists see heart problems everywhere. They wouldn't be cardiologists without their resonance with the subject of love, because they would not notice heart diseases and would not have an interest in it in the first place. Once they resolve those issues, they might change careers. The word issue here is not meant to have a negative connotation. We can label our issues positive or negative if we wish, but these labels are not intrinsic to the subject.

Two different cardiologists may seek out different lessons about the same disease. These doctors also mirror our society. On some level we all resonate with these issues, otherwise our society would not produce cardiologists in the first place. Once they learn their specific lessons, they ultimately promote a resolution of these interweaving personal and collective issues for many of us. In other words, once this is accomplished, part of the task has symbolically been completed for humanity as a whole.

We have been educated to look outside ourselves for answers to problems. By doing this, we can fall into the trap of blaming circumstances and assuming the role of victimhood, which is as old as humanity. Adam and Eve blamed the serpent for their act of transgression. By not taking responsibility they gave away their power, dissolved oneness and created polarities. Their unity with the Creator split into duality: inside – outside, good – bad, I – the other. Through this they helped define and give birth to the world of duality we know today. Adam and Eve symbolize us, still looking elsewhere for answers about who to love and who to blame, about good or bad, how to act, what to feel, and who will heal us.

Consequently, our medical establishment is concerned with suppressing symptoms, creating dependencies on technology and treating bodies like machines. We were not trained to heal the internal issues that cause external manifestations. When we treat a symptom rather than the underlying issue that triggered the symptom, the same symptom often appears later with increased intensity, or in a different form.

Sometimes a new symptom or disease may occur and complicate the matter. In our hospitals, virtually nobody except a priest is willing to ask how a patient is feeling on a deep spiritual level. What is the patient's purpose in life? How does he see his life relationships, emotions, his past and future, his unfulfilled desires? How does he feel about his disease and symptoms; why is there a need to experience them? What kind of person does he truly long to become?

Admittedly, the majority of patients would have vague, unclear answers to these questions. They may not be willing to take a closer look at themselves and prefer an outside quick-fix. This quick-fix syndrome is a clear mirror of what is happening within us. However, as more and more patients are seeking out healing on the deeper levels of human nature, inevitably, science and modern medicine will follow.

Cause versus Correlation (Heart Disease and Cholesterol)

The modern scientific approach to illness and disease is focused on studies and statistical correlations. Even though the correlations may be significant, the real causes and sources of these diseases are not easy to establish. Medical books contain long lists of what they consider to be causes of disease, but all the lists in the world cannot answer exactly why you got the disease and not someone else with the same diet, weight, exercise and smoking habits, or why you got it at this particular point in your life and how your symptoms correlate with other events in your life. They don't tell you why people with the healthiest lifestyles in the world can become ill.

Statisticians know that correlations and associations might have different causes. Sometimes an association may work for different reasons than we actually see. An association A-B may have a common source C on a level that we cannot perceive (see **Figure 5**) and we may think that A causes B when in fact C is the cause for both of them. For example, if lots of robberies occur during the night, that does not mean that the night is the cause of the robberies. Trying to reduce the nighttime with artificial

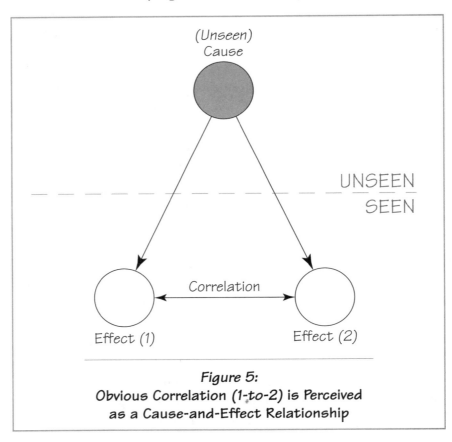

Figure 5:
Obvious Correlation (1-to-2) is Perceived
as a Cause-and-Effect Relationship

light to reduce the robbery rate may work to some extent, but it does not remove the actual cause of robbery. In the same way, we can say with a fairly high degree of confidence that it is not cholesterol, fat, lack of exercise, smoking, drinking and indulging that cause certain diseases. These elements are merely correlations, i.e. they appear in conjunction with disease.

Cholesterol has been blamed for many health problems. There is much money and politics involved in this issue and interests are high to make you believe so. If cholesterol causes heart problems, then why is it that half of the heart attack patients have normal levels of cholesterol? It is true that many individuals with a higher level of cholesterol are at increased risk for heart attack, but so are people who snore or speak English. The fact that half of the heart disease subjects have higher level of cholesterol does not necessarily mean that cholesterol is the source of the heart attack. There may simply be a high correlation between the kind of behavior that generates both fat and heart disease. It may also mean that a deteriorating condition of the heart could produce a higher level of cholesterol. There is in fact a correlation between fat cravings and emotional denials that create heart disease. Eating fat does not directly create heart disease, it may just make you throw up.

Cholesterol is a kind of fat that is as essential to our bodies as are vitamins – and probably more important. Without cholesterol, life as we know it would not be possible. All our cell membranes contain cholesterol, and half of our body's hormones, including the sex hormones, are made of cholesterol. Seventy-five percent of your brain is cholesterol. In fact, cholesterol is so crucial to life that nature provided a mechanism to make sure that we will never lack it. The liver manufactures cholesterol continuously and insures that the cholesterol supply is never based on sole ingestion from external sources. More than two thirds of it is manufactured inside the body according to our needs, while less than one third is taken from our diet. This is why people with normal diets may still have a high level of cholesterol. It is known that cholesterol is beneficial for the body and the current theory postulates that only oxidized cholesterol may play a negative role. But even that may be a correlation with our life patterns.

Everything around us exists to help us in some way, and cholesterol is no exception. Let us try to understand how cholesterol may be helpful to us. Millions of times a year the heart beats to pump blood through the blood vessels. If, for whatever reason, these vessels lose their elasticity, they can develop cracks due to rigidity. The body in its wisdom sends cholesterol to the rescue and patches these cracks with a glue-like band-aid. In order for the patch to stay in place, it needs to become oxidized and calcified – in other words, it has to be transformed into a semipermanent patch. However, when the patch itself becomes rigid, a new crack may develop. In this way, the body plasters itself with patch over patch, until the blood vessel becomes almost blocked. The more rigid your arteries are, the more patches you need, so your body will manufacture more and more cholesterol. Overwhelmed by the body's constant demand for cholesterol, the liver goes into overdrive, trying to meet the need.

High cholesterol in your blood is a sign of rigid arteries, symbolizing a rigid way of life. It is this rigidity, this refusal to feel and flow, that ultimately causes heart disease. As you can see, cholesterol might be nothing more than an innocent bystander that came into the picture to help.

An elevated level of cholesterol in the blood also symbolically reveals two emotional issues: An increased need for joy (reflected by narrowed arteries), and a need for emotional protection against the lack of joy that translates into fatty deposits inside the arteries). Reducing cholesterol by medication works to a point, but has nothing to do with healing the disease. The emotional denial that creates the craving for fat is also what contributes to heart disease and high blood pressure. If someone refuses to feel, depending upon what the refusal is about, this person can contract heart disease, high blood pressure or diabetes. They are all associated with fat, but it is not the fat that caused it. You can be as thin as possible and still get heart disease.

Fat and Symbols (Diet)

If we keep in mind that we are not victims, and that everything around mirrors our thought patterns, then every disease and craving is helping us see our issues. If we can consciously realize why there is a need for a craving or disease and how it mirrors our thought patterns and emotional status, we can eliminate those issues much faster and release the need to be sick. We may crave fats, salt or sugar. There might be an underlying need for them because they help us deal with the issues involved. If we are able to resolve the issues that communicate to us through the craving, that specific craving will disappear.

Fats help us deal with anger, help us process emotions and life circumstances that made anger manifest. Sugar is an artificial substitute for love and sweetness in our life. Salt helps us flow, let go of unnecessary burdens and deal with fears. The presence of fats in the stomach triggers a release of bile from the gallbladder. Bile in turn is necessary for further absorption of fats. Fats are then assimilated and distributed to the body cells where they act as mental and emotional insulators. Fats protect us from the mental and emotional onslaught of the circumstances that made us angry. This insulation gives processing time to the liver. Depending on how well the liver processes the situation, more or less bile is formed.

It is known that anger elicits contractions of the gallbladder and is also known that a discharge of bile increases the liver function.

Two important conclusions are emerging from this: One is that we need fats when we are angry, because the fat acts as a mental and emotional shield that protects us from anger and helps us clear it. Secondly, the fat content in our body is not relevant as a direct cause of disease. Instead of being so concerned about the fat content of the food , we had better find and resolve the issue that makes us crave the fat in the first place.

Any craving is a reflection (symbolic mirror) of an issue. The craving is there to communicate something to us; it is a messenger, not an enemy. I suggest we listen to all cravings, because they serve a purpose.

Life events are not here to defeat us. We manifest them for the purpose of stepping forward on our spiritual path. May we listen and honor them.

Symbolic Complications (Diabetes)

Individuals have a desire to experience love and harmony. Deep inside our body there is an organ that symbolically helps us assimilate this feeling of love and harmony: the pancreas. The pancreas secretes juices that facilitate the symbolic absorption of the sweetness of life. Specialized cells in this organ help us assimilate experiences at a deep, cellular and spiritual level.

Insulin, secreted by the pancreas, assists sugars in crossing the cell membrane, to be symbolically absorbed into the basic structures of our beings. Our need to ingest sweets depends on how removed we feel from love and harmony. You may have noticed that when people feel lonely and not loved enough they eat a lot of sweets. When they feel loved and happy they don't need the substitutes. Our children crave love. If we give them generous amounts of affection and caring, their craving for candies will diminish. Indulgence in sweets also represents a sweet escape from daily meals (ongoing experiences).

Chocolate is a symbolic substitute for physical affection. It is solid (physical) and contains sugar and caffeine – love and excitement, the emotions related to sexuality. Since it does not belong to any of the food families, chocolate also symbolizes an exciting, sweet escape from daily experiences. Vanilla, the sweet taste of mother's desserts, is a symbol for family. A craving for chocolate or vanilla ice cream may represent a need to soothe specific desires related to issues of sex or family.

People who feel hurt by circumstances may subconsciously decide not to experience the sweetness of life anymore. For example, when a spouse dies, the remaining one may feel shocked, lonely or perhaps guilty, and subconsciously decide that sweetness is not worth experiencing anymore. Consequently, less and less sugar enters this person's body cells.

This mental/emotional pattern translates into a complex set of symptoms and afflictions which, in medical terms, is called *diabetes mellitus*. It can manifest in many different ways, but generally crystallizes around a typical group of symptoms and behaviors.

Diabetics eat a lot. Food is symbolic for ingesting life in its richness and fullness. Rich food can become a substitute for life experiences that seem less than satisfying. Diabetics often drink a lot of water (a symbolic need to absorb emotions), but these emotions are ultimately denied and the water is eliminated through the bladder as quickly as it came in. These patients also eliminate sugars through their urine (they reject the sweetness). For a better understanding of the diabetes complications, please see **Table 4**.

In viewing this list, please remember that nobody is to be blamed or made wrong for having a disease. Ultimately, disease is an indication that we are choosing a hard way to learn and grow in life.

> ### Table 4:
> ### Symbolic Complications – Diabetes mellitus
>
> | | SYMBOLIC CAUSE: | SYMBOLIC EFFECT: |
> |---|---|---|
> | 1. | Refusal to see harmony | Eye problems (retinopathy) |
> | 2. | Narrow flow of life | Atherosclerosis |
> | 3. | Anger toward life | Vasculitis |
> | 4. | Refusal to receive or give love | Heart problems |
> | 5. | Indecision | Foot problems |
> | 6. | General anger | Inflammations (infections) |
> | 7. | Relationship issues | Autonomic neuropathy |
> | 8. | Low self-image | Skin problems |
> | 9. | Denial of emotions, feelings | Sensory neuropathy |
> | 10. | Helplessness, hopelessness | Nervous problems, coma |
> | 11. | Lack of joy and vitality | Anemia |
> | 12. | Feeling unsupported, angry | Bone diseases, osteomyelitis |
> | 13. | Lack of flexibility | Joint problems |
> | 14. | Refusal to assimilate events | Digestive problems |
> | 15. | Fears, inability to let go | Kidney problems |
> | 16. | Holding onto emotions | Bladder problems |

Also, different body parts have varying symbolic associations for different people. It is the same with dreams – the general symbolism is valid, but we need to take into account each person's uniquely individual dimension. It would be good to stop and think for a while about yourself, to understand your particular association with certain organs or illnesses.

Cancers and Symbols

Symbolically, cancer represents an emotional issue that is eating us from the inside out. Cancer is usually a red flag signaling that a hidden aspect within ourselves desperately wants to be acknowledged and loved. We're dealing with something we have not yet learned to accept as ours; something deprived of love that is spreading like a weed in order to be noticed. This need can be so great that it takes over a person's life.

When unexpressed and unexperienced emotions limit our purpose and expression on this planet, we may be challenged by this disease. Cancer, like everything else, is consciousness projected into matter. Each time we perceive our surroundings as something to be casually used and eaten up, we behave like a cancerous cell. We actually manufacture at least one cancerous cell every time we think or behave that way. The more we are caught up in such thoughts, the more we are at risk of developing cancer.

The key to understanding disease is to remain appreciative and grateful for each and every experience, realizing that it is but a mirror of us. If we allow ourselves to flow with the currents of life without blame or resistance, we may never experience cancer.

The organs affected by cancer are symbolically representative of the issue that needs to be addressed. For example, the multitude of cancers of the sexual organs that we see in modern culture reflects our confusion around sexuality. Risk factors, such as smoking, toxins and carcinogens, are likely to be just associations to cancer. Smoking has a particularly strong symbolic significance: We are attempting to hide behind a smoke screen to avoid new inspirations and keep at a distance from the intensity of life's experiences.

Joints and Symbols

Joints are symbolic of flexibility and ease of movement in the body, mind and emotions. Their level of efficiency is a good indicator of the way we adjust to changing circumstances. We may feel stiffness or rigidity; that symbolically translates into a lack of flexibility in our attitudes and difficulty to bend with life circumstances. Feelings of guilt, criticism, skepticism and despair can symbolically correspond to feelings of pain, rigidity, stiffness and disjointedness.

Figure 6 describes the flow of vital energy through the body. When we raise our hands to the sky, energy flows in through the hand, moves down through the body and exits from the feet as it enters the earth, thus establishing a connection between above and below; between the sky and the earth. The first junction point within this current is marked by our wrists, the first major joint in the energy pathway. Wrists correspond to the respiratory system and lungs.

The elbow, the second gateway, corresponds to the circulatory system and the heart. We begin to process the energy when it reaches the shoulders, which therefore correspond to the liver. The current then flows to the hips where we symbolically absorb and digest what is needed before channeling the rest of it down to the knees and ankles, which correspond to the elimination system. The elimination system helps circulate and recycle the energy back to nature in order to complete the circuit.

Each joint mirrors the degree of flexibility and support we feel in life. Since ancient times, arthritis and arthrosis have been correlated with criticism and judgment. What else are criticism and judgments, but an inability to see a different point of view, to allow, to accept and to flow? When we stick to seeing things our way, we are stuck. Symbolically and literally, this can translate into arthrosis and joint problems.

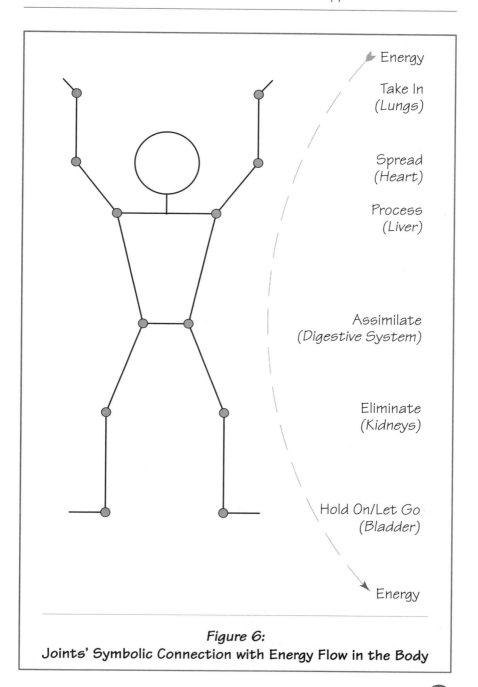

Figure 6:
Joints' Symbolic Connection with Energy Flow in the Body

Table 5: Joints and Their Associated Symbolic Function		
JOINT	ORGAN	FUNCTION
1. Wrists	Lungs/large intestine	Absorbing/releasing
2. Elbows	Heart/small intestine	Circulation/spreading
3. Shoulders	Liver/gallbladder	Processing/timing
4. Hips	Stomach/spleen/ pancreas	Digesting/integrating
5. Knees/ankles	Kidney/bladder	Holding/releasing

Symbolic Symptoms (The Common Cold)

The messages we receive through our symptoms are not vague and abstract, but purposeful, detailed and specific. They are, in fact, the body's way of communicating. Once we learn how to interpret the symbolic language, we can honor the body's requests, and symptoms will disappear. If we don't get the messages and their scope remains unfulfilled, then the symptoms worsen, become chronic or get smart and develop into something else. Symptoms exist to catch our attention so that we change, accept and love ourselves. In order to under-stand how minor symptoms operate in the context of a disease let's analyze an example of a common cold, a so-called respira-tory tract infection.

Our subject is John, 25 years old, working hard and feeling pressured to work even harder. Because of many parties, travels and various hobbies, he is perpetually short of cash and works on weekends to make extra money. He just split up with his girl friend. He doesn't really feel understood by his mother, even though he knows that she loves him. Today, he woke up feeling strange and a bit dizzy. (His subconscious is telling him that there is just too much pressure, but John doesn't realize this.) During his regular morning exercises, he finds that he is a little weaker than usual. (The body needs rest.) "What is going on with me?" he thinks. "I'll take a vitamin or an aspirin and everything will be okay." He takes both, feels a little better and gets ready for work. He coughs a couple of times at the thought of work, but doesn't even notice it. (We know that coughing means he is rejecting the idea of going to work.)

John pushes through the minor symptoms of weakness and goes to work because he feels he needs the money. On the way out, he cuts his right thumb on the door lock. (This symbolically translates into guilt and worry about the obstinate, intellectual control process that tries to overcome the instinctual feelings of letting go and staying home.) A small amount of blood is gushing from the cut (signaling joy and vitality that are leaking as the result of the logical decisions.) He puts on a bandaid and goes to work. After a while, his throat becomes tingly and achy.

The developing sore throat represents anger toward not expressing his needs, not acknowledging them and not communicating. It hurts to swallow because it feels uncomfortable to assimilate new experiences. John keeps on working. After a while, his nose becomes stuffy and fills with secretions (he doesn't want to take in more experiences at work).

John's whole body is saying, "Give me a break; slow down and take off work now." He is resisting: "No, I'm not listening to you; I will stay here and work."

Nausea sets in (which symbolically indicates an unwillingness to assimilate the experience). His throat is becoming worse. After a while, he feels dizzier and has chills (he feels out of

Table 6:
Symbolic Symptoms: The Common Cold (John's Case)

SYMPTOM:	SYMBOLIC ASSOCIATION:
1. Cough	Resistance, rejection
2. Right thumb	Logic, intellect, acceptance
3. Pain	Denial, refusal of an experience
4. Hemorrhage	Leaking of vitality and joy
5. Throat	Communication & expression
6. Sore throat	Suppressing (swallowing) anger
7. Swallowing	Acceptance of new experiences
8. Stuffy or runny nose	Emotional refusal of experience
9. Nausea	Physical rejection
10. Dizziness	Refusal to focus or be present in the moment
11. Chills	Trying to shake off an unpleasant experience
12. Fever	Generalized anger
13. Short, sharp pain	Short, sharp denial

control and wants to rid himself of this experience.) He doesn't want to be there and is considering going home versus staying at work. He realizes that he has a fever (signaling generalized anger about the situation).

He is thinking, "Why does this happen to me now, when I need the money?" At this exact moment, a brief, sharp pain shoots through his lower back (indicating his momentary distrust in the ability of life to support him in all his needs).

After an hour passes by, his boss finally notices that John is not feeling well, and sends him home after a short conversation. On the way home, John realizes that his throat is not as bad as it was.

His feelings were expressed, but his throat is still sore. He is confused and cannot think clearly. He needs to take a break from worrying and too much thinking. His coughing has intensified (as he symbolically rejects and resists this situation). It seems that the only thing he can do at this time is to go home and rest.

After two days of bed rest and nurturing by his mother, John wakes up feeling energized, healthy and ready to go to work. His overworked body has manifested a short disease in order to give him a break and stop thinking for a while. Once he has received the rest he needed, he is able to return to work with more energy, greater health and a clearer mind.

People generally know the cause of their illness, consciously or subconsciously. They just choose not to respond to the messages of the illness, because it would require inconvenient changes. Many patients remain in denial of an unhealthy situation and choose not to change it, because they feel it is either too difficult or there is too much at stake. These denials can persist for years. It is indeed challenging to question one's habits, belief system, past actions, etc.

Symptoms and diseases become amplified until sooner or later a change is being forced through circumstances – which are, in fact, a mirror of our internal processing. It is not the weather or the government or some mean virus that forces us, it is ourselves who choose to force the issue.

How do we know what our issues are? In general, the situation that we want to avoid the most tends to be the one that needs the most attention.

It is very important not to be put down by the interpretation of an illness. Illness is a tool that can be used creatively. Once we learn to work with it instead of against it, the internal conflicts will disappear. Symbolic messages are reflective mirrors designed to help us recognize the divinity inside.

Part IV
CELLS AND PERCEPTION

❖ ❖ ❖

"You are creating yourself everyday.
Seek therefore not to find out who you are
but to determine who you want to be."

❖ ❖ ❖

Focus on Disease

Now, that we have a broad understanding of symbolic disease, it is time to apply that understanding in a practical way.

Remember that whatever we focus on, receives energy. The meaning of a focus is a place of applied attention where energies converge (see **Figure 7**). Quantum physics teaches that the act of observation affects the subject of observation. So, our focus

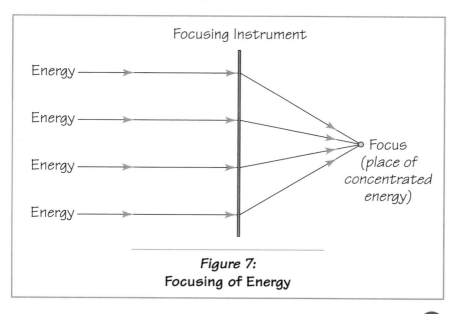

Focusing Instrument

Energy

Energy

Energy

Energy

Focus
(place of
concentrated
energy)

Figure 7:
Focusing of Energy

determines the nature of reality. By changing our focus, we automatically change our reality and our experiences.

This concept of focusing is not just a beautiful philosophical idea, but has very practical applications in life. Symbolically and literally, when we focus on something we send energy at a high, invisible frequency to the object involved. For example, when we attend a rock concert, the energies of many people are focused on the protagonist. Invisible strands of energy link the singer with the audience. The singer may feel this energy and experience a state of energetic high, which can be extremely addictive. At the end, the applause serves to energetically disconnect each individual from the singer's energy field. The more intense the emotions and the focus, the longer and stronger the applause.

Let's say we walk out of a movie theater after an intensely gripping movie. Our stirred emotions tend to linger for a while and we may not feel totally present. No applause was involved. Realize how different we feel with and without applause. By clapping the hands we refocus our attention back to the immediate physical vicinity.

Whatever receives our focus, receives importance, grows and amplifies. We may focus on beauty, we may focus on love or we may focus on fear. This is not wishful thinking; it is a concrete physical law. The only difference is that you don't hear about it in school.

Mainstream medicine focuses on the physical aspect of the human being. The three nonphysical aspects of our personality – emotional, mental and spiritual – are not receiving much attention. Again, this is not to be labeled as good or bad; it is simply a reflection of what our present society chooses to focus on.

However, time has come to consider the human being as more complex, more humane and more divine. We can learn to balance difficult aspects of our personality by understanding them rather than fighting them. The physical mechanism of our body is a solidification and a lower vibrational aspect of more subtle thought patterns. By focusing solely on the physical level, we may become aware of only physical experiences, but the hidden feeling of missing something important becomes overwhelming. By focusing only on mental or spiritual aspects, we also forget that the physical body is in fact spirit in flesh and the temple of the soul. Together, the four aspects form a unique whole, that has a spiritual journey as its ultimate purpose.

It is worthwhile to detach ourselves momentarily from the analytical separative perspective and embrace the whole. It is like a shift to a satellite view of the earth: borders disappear in favor of relationship and cooperation, and the sense of being human is strengthened. Someone said that problems can be resolved only from a perspective higher than the one in which they were created. By changing the focus to a more unifying perspective, we can add meaning to life while enjoying all four aspects of our human condition.

These days are marked by many medical subspecialties and other branches of healing that use a more holistic approach. Remember that acupuncture or eating natural foods are not by themselves holistic medicine, but they each contribute a piece to the total picture. The symbolic approach to disease is intended as a step in understanding ourselves. There is still a long way to that holistic place we intend to reach, but every beginning is less than perfect. What counts is our intention – and our focus.

Cells and How They Work

Let's explore the human physiology in greater depth to discover how the theory of symbolic associations can be applied at the cellular level. The correlations that reveal themselves at this very fundamental layer of life are utterly fascinating. Since the cellular processes are somewhat removed from general public knowledge, I will try to keep it simple and easy to understand.

A cell is a tiny building block of the body comparable in appearance and function to the whole organism. We can think of the cell as a miniature representation of the body, having its own symbolic counterparts of the major body structures. Every cell has its own skin (membrane), head (nucleolus), heart (nucleus), circulatory system (endoplasmic reticulum), liver (mitochondria), digestive system (lysosomes), skeleton (microtubules) and so on (see **Figure 8**).

Human cells are grouped together within the tissues and organs. All organs, systems and cells operate according to our intrinsic internal order, share duties and uphold communication with each other. One can say that cells, tissues and organs function together like an advanced society.

Bacteria and Viruses

Bacteria, on the other hand, function as single cells, separated from one another by thick walls. Their primitive structure

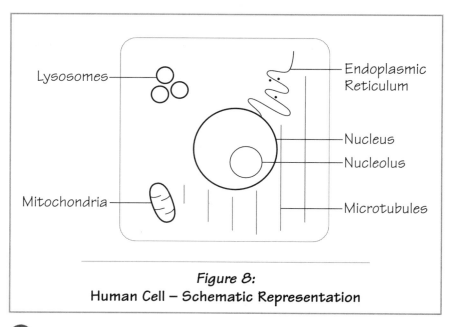

Figure 8:
Human Cell – Schematic Representation

contains only a rudimentary circular DNA and no nucleus. This pattern symbolically indicates a lack of heart value; a lack of integration, higher purpose and insight into the inherent intelligence of the whole organism. These organisms share no intrinsic order and don't help each other. Some of them even diffuse dangerous substances or toxins (feelings) into their environment. An obvious parallel can be drawn to the behavior of a person engaged in thoughts of victimhood, isolation, anger, etc. Bacteria are symbolic of trapped feelings and primitive self-limited behavior due to a limited or distorted perception of the environment.

For example, let us explain what happens on the battlefield of an infection: In the blood there are specialized cells called neutrophils, in charge of maintaining law and order, and specialized in helping all other cells. They are the policemen on the streets (in the blood vessels). In case of an emergency, a general alarm is sounded in the whole body which immediately mobilizes a massive rush of police force to the affected area. Many of these policemen may die, and reinforcements are sent to the site. These new policemen appear together with veterans in higher numbers on the streets, armed with powerful weapons called enzymes (promoters of change) that are capable of breaking down and dissolving solid tissue.

These policemen are trained to move in with full force, unafraid to die for their cause (your health), and many do die quickly. However, the inherent intelligence of the body has also provided us with longer lasting firefighters and scavengers called macrophages, whose purpose is to cleanse and restore the tissue. Sometimes their work is sufficient to restore an affected area to health, but when there is residual danger, they call up the environmentalists (lymphocytes) for help. After determining the extent of the damage, these lymphocytes organize strategies and design safety zones around the damage area. Next come the builders (fibroblasts) who construct these safety areas. These areas of safety usually contain lots of environmental and scavenger security officers in charge of supervising all activities. When this level of security stays in place for an extended period of time, we are actually dealing with a chronic infection.

Bacteria are symbolic primitive aspects of ourselves, primitive caricatures of our emotional reactions that we use when we feel threatened. Bacteria have strong cell walls or capsules (strong defense systems). Symbolically speaking, they do not have a good concept of their purpose, which is reflected in the fact that they don't have organized nucleoli and nuclei (they don't have a head or heart – they don't think or feel). They are always hungry and multiply like crazy. They stick together and like to be where it is warm and moist. From their home base, they usually launch attacks with different substances called toxins. These creatures have an exaggerated sense of self-preservation because they feel threatened. Their strong cell wall or capsule indicates this preoccupation with self defense.

Bacteria do not become part of us unless we feel threatened. If we don't feel threatened, there is usually no bacteria in our body, with the exception of those on our skin (a mirror of defensive attitudes) and upper digestive tract. Sometimes we believe that we may be threatened by people or circumstances around us, or by what we may accidentally absorb. Because these are only potentially threatening circumstances that are not actually happening, bacteria in these situations have a round shape (symbolic of yet unmanifest circumstances). No other body part (except the upper airways which are also part of the digestive system) normally contains bacteria.

The characteristics of bacteria can teach us much about basic human behavior. For example, we were taught many lessons in politeness and good manners for the day-to-day situations. However, as soon as we feel threatened, we forget the niceties and switch to our defense mode. Primitive survival instincts of defense (attack, violence, food and sex) appear dominant when we feel threatened. If you happened to survive a shipwreck on a remote island, needing to fight for your life with animals or indigent tribes, you would most likely drop your present way of being. The only difference, then, would be that you would accept this way of life openly so you would not manifest an infection.

Bacteria are primitive caricatures of our basic emotional reactions to threat. Their microbiological behavior varies according to the circumstances; they may be slimy or aggressive, hide behind a hard shell or spread poisons. So, they can easily be seen as miniscule organisms that mimic human behavior. For example, if we isolate ourselves out of fear that something might happen, we will manifest bacteria with strong cell walls in our body. If we spread intrigues and (counter-)attack our environment, we manifest a kind of bacteria that spreads powerful toxins in the body.

We are all familiar with the widespread belief that we catch illnesses from sick people. Those who get away without catching something think they must have been lucky. However, a sick person only mirrors our own attitudes or thought patterns and acts as a warning signal to indicate that we will get sick if we don't change. In fact, by mirroring us, they do us a favor.

When we wear red glasses, everything looks red. A society looking through the glasses of victimhood will naturally see victims everywhere. When the color of the glasses is changed, perspectives and perceptions change accordingly. From this point of view, bacteria are not bad by themselves, any more than a mirror image is.

Antibiotic treatments work sometimes, and sometimes they don't. By sincerely accepting a treatment, we relinquish our defenses and surrender to help and change. In fact, the way many antibiotics work is by dissolving bacterial defenses.

Symbolically, these antibiotics only work if we let down our defenses. Antibiotics can have lasting effects if we are willing to heal the issue and accept the change. Otherwise, people develop resistance to antibiotics and the dis-ease continues undisturbed.

Viruses look like abstract sculptures or thought patterns, and this is exactly what they symbolize. They are lifeless elements with no intention or action of their own. What we call live viruses in scientific terms, are complete viral structures, such as a whole cube, for example. Dead viruses are fragments of an initial, complete virus structure, like pieces of a cube. However, because viruses have no metabolism, don't breathe or consume energy, they are not alive in any true sense of the word.

The most dangerous knife cannot enter your body unless somebody pushes it. Lifeless elements, like thought patterns and viruses, cannot attack us. The point here is that cells are actively accepting a virus. In light of this, the idea of fighting against a virus does not make sense.

The human body is a manifestation of consciousness, and each cell is a materialization of a thought form. We really create ourselves through our own personal and collective thoughts. Thoughts of a similar nature blend together to form living beliefs that influence our organs to function according to those beliefs. If thoughts are in harmony with each other and respectful of the surroundings, then we develop tissues that operate harmoniously. Small thoughts of isolation manifest as sensations (feelings) of isolation that are physically projected into bacteria. If our hidden and repressed thoughts revolve around taking advantage of someone or something, we might even manifest cancerous cells. Remember that the interpretation we want to attach to these processes differ from person to person. There is always a positive reason or silver lining to everything we consider to be negative. Let me explain the positive implications of cancer.

Cancer Cells

To understand cancer cells, we have to know something about cell shape. The shape of a cell is contingent upon its function. A well differentiated cell has a well defined task which requires a well defined cell shape that is adapted to its particular purpose. The more differentiated and purposeful the task, the less rounded the cell shape. An undifferentiated cell has undifferentiated unmanifested potential with a corresponding circular shape. An ovum (egg cell), for example, contains the virtually limitless potential for the formation of all the cells of a new human being. All possibilities are inherent within this cell, giving it its characteristic round shape. In terms of symbolic representation, we can say that the circle represents unmanifested perfection, whereas the square stands for manifest finite perfection (see **Figure 9**).

Cancerous cells lack a well defined purpose and tend to be circular, as well. In fact, there is a direct correlation between their lack of differentiation and the extent of their potential to grow. So, the silver lining of cancer is unmistakable: the undifferentiated, limitless potential of cancer cells are an indication of the person's unlimited potential for hope, change, growth and evolution through this disease that is so feared by society. (More on cancer later.) For a better understanding of cell functions, see **Figure 8** (page 92) and **Figure 11** (page 103).

DNA and RNA

Let us now investigate the mechanics of a thought manifesting into a concrete physical cell. The internal health status of a cell reflects our internal physical health, whereas the condition of a cell's outer environment symbolically corresponds to that of our surroundings. Thoughts arise from the innermost center of our being at the mental level, which is represented by the cell nucleolus.

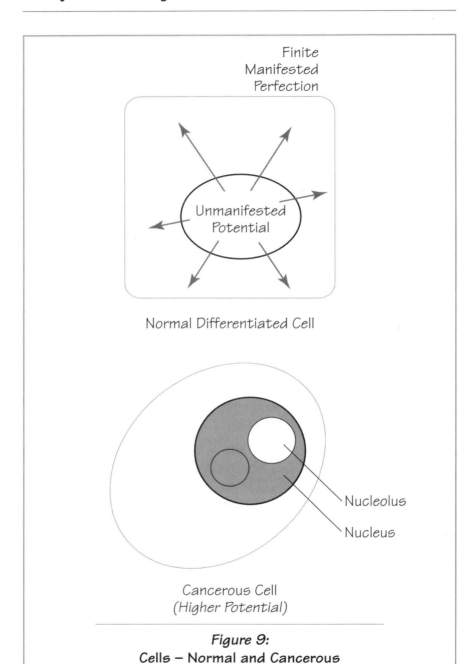

Finite
Manifested
Perfection

Unmanifested
Potential

Normal Differentiated Cell

Nucleolus

Nucleus

Cancerous Cell
(Higher Potential)

Figure 9:
Cells – Normal and Cancerous

Within this nucleolus, DNA tells RNA what to create and how to proceed.

This selective process is responsible for integrating, classifying and evaluating our life experiences. The nucleolus then manufactures ribosomes (substances that pass from the nucleolus into the bigger nucleus) which spread DNA information through a liquid (emotional medium) and from there to the whole cell.

Ribosomes further manufacture proteins which are the building blocks of organic matter and life. Proteins correspond to physical matter; they symbolize mental and emotional processes that lower their vibration in order to manifest as physical matter. Thus, we can say that at the cellular level (which, again, is a small mirror of the whole organism), thoughts proceed from the mental realm to the emotional realm and only then do they finally reveal themselves physically. This is the hermetic law of nature: As above, so below.

The larger the nucleus and nucleolus in proportion to the body, the younger the cell is considered to be (the same principle applies to humans). Young cells have a higher potential of activity, which shapes rounder physical forms.

A closer look at the characteristic shape of the DNA strands (**Figure 10**) unveils a series of highly suggestive symbolic correlations. As we have seen before, DNA chains are a powerful symbol that represents the supposed and agreed upon blueprint of our destiny. RNA is a symbol of the way we work out this destiny. In other words, the way the RNA works shows our capacity to accept or change a DNA symbolic destiny. The characteristic double helicoidal spiral shape of the DNA strand symbolizes growth and unfoldment by successive and cumulative experiences. Memories from the past are contained in the present and somehow repeated, providing background and support for future experiences. The double helix is an expression of a specific past and an indication of what will be experienced next. It is a continuous longing, not yet unfolded, operating in specific cycles.

Each cycle or coil of DNA contains ten bases or building blocks. Ten is the number of infinity manifesting into individuality. These

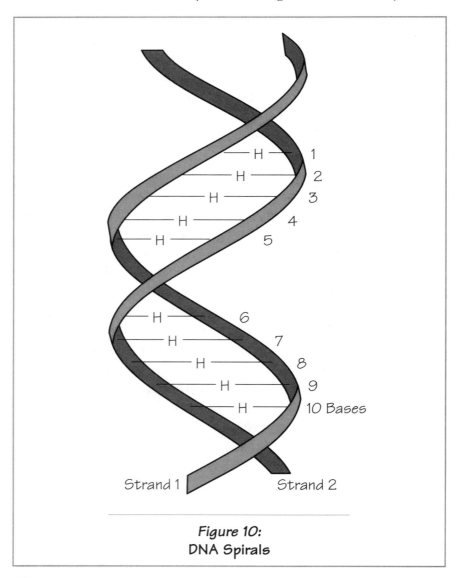

Figure 10:
DNA Spirals

building blocks can be subdivided into five different types – three plus two. They form the double helix with two parallel chains. The two related chains are held together by hydrogen (H) bonds and have the power to split apart into two complementary chains, suggestive of the physical duality (male/female, up/down, in/out) of the physical world. Numeric symbolism teaches us that five is the number of life, whereas two (the number of strands) symbolizes multiplicity, the power of moving from a static state to a dynamic state, and the power to generate form within oneself. For a deeper understanding of the DNA structure please look at **Figure 10**.

Cells and Their Channels

Within the cellular membrane of a cell there are channels that form connections with the environment. It is through these channels that the cells interact with their surroundings. They represent the mechanism of our personal interactions with the environment. The symbolic implications are clear: These channels are already in place, which indicates that we are going to experience our world according to our pre-established, pre-determined connections.

We cannot have a certain experience unless we possess a potential predisposition toward that experience. For example, we cannot have the experience of climbing a mountain if we are not willing to climb one. We cannot have an intense experience of a religious celebration in a remote country if we don't have cultural connections to that culture which predispose us for this type of experience.

Cellular channels mirror our potential for assimilating expe-riences. They represent a connection and an opening. When we are open to change, these channels are opened. Change repre-sents a threat to the currently established identity because changing means giving up something from the inside and taking in something from the outside, otherwise information cannot be ex-changed. Communication is impossible without change! Through change, we symbolically increase our vulnerability, but also our power.

Ultimately, change represents a step toward oneness. Cell relationships with their surroundings symbolize this, as well. There are channels in the cellular membrane that make the connection to the outside. We can only perceive and experience something if we symbolically connect to that object. The process of perception symbolically indicates a connection between inside and outside. This connection requires a definite change from our normal, isolated (inside oriented) perception of an individual. Remember that our cells are made of thought patterns that model us (as above, so below).

Why is change so important? The need for change within living tissue is stimulated by the desire for a state of balance, which is achieved through the maintenance of an optimum quantity of elements inside and outside of the cells. When a connection to the outside takes place, the old state is disrupted and the new dynamic balance takes over. Needed substances from the outside are absorbed internally, while substances from the inside are dispensed outward. See **Figure 11** for a better understanding of cell symbolism and cell channels.

This game of exchange is played by the elements of sodium and potassium. Sodium (salt) is a symbolic earth element that exists outside of us, in the oceans and the earth and, not coincidentally, outside and around the cells. Sodium keeps the emotions flowing and balances them with the needs of the cells. When one feels strongly affected by external events and needs to stabilize the emotions, the body responds with a craving for salt. The symbolic explanation is that, in times of danger, we tend not to listen to our emotions. These emotions are minimized and repressed because at this time our focus is on surviving or coping mechanisms. Only when the overwhelming factor has passed, can we again allow the natural flow of emotions.

Salt then acts as a facilitator to free the emotional flow, which is much needed to restore the equilibrium. Once inside the body, salt makes us thirsty, since it encourages liquids (representing emotions) to flow in and then out of the body. Elimination of excess water is done easily if there are no other blocking mechanisms. By increasing the input and output of fluids in the body, salt helps the free flow of water, which is symbolic of the free flow of emotions. Salt cravings help reconnect us with an emotionally balanced state. In other words, an increased concentration of

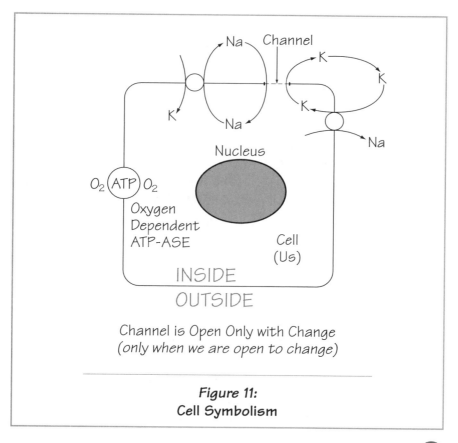

Channel is Open Only with Change
(only when we are open to change)

Figure 11:
Cell Symbolism

sodium in the cell surroundings attracts more water which is then eliminated by the kidneys in an effort to help the system maintain an emotional balance. One can see that it is important to understand the mechanisms of cravings in order to appreciate the underlying wisdom and respond appropriately to maintain our physical and emotional health.

Cells and Perception

The perceiver vibrates on a same wavelength as the object of perception. We just explored the sodium and potassium interplay across the cell membrane, which makes possible the exchange of information across the cell membrane. All signals – all perceptions – can ultimately be traced back to a form of sodium and potassium interplay inside and outside the cell. This exchange constitutes the very basis of a nervous stimulus. Depending upon the specificity (nerves themselves may be sensitive to only one color or only one sound, etc.), a cell may be sensitive to a wide range of stimuli or only to a few groups of select signals.

To see, we need light; we need a burning fire somewhere. Light particles emanate from a source of light and move through different media (the air stands for the mental layer, and eye liquids signify emotional elements) before they are received by our internal eye. Different wavelengths of light resonate with different vision cells according to the vibrational frequencies that the vision cells are attuned to. Symbolically, vision cells are receptive only to those spiritual messages that match the receptivity and willingness of the person to perceive. The light or fire that is required for vision to occur is a symbolic representation of our spiritual and internal fire which is required in order for us to exist at all.

Vision is a feedback loop. The things that we see are mirroring our beliefs back to us. The world around us is nothing but a projection of our own spiritually induced manifestations into the physical realm. Sometimes, if we don't feel ready to accept this symbolic feedback, we may choose to decrease our vision to avoid seeing what lies ahead of us.

The sense of hearing works in a similar manner. Hearing requires sound, which is produced by a movement (vibration). Every pitch, tone and rhythm evokes a specific emotion. Similarly to light, the sound messages pass through the air (the mental level) and liquids (internal ear fluids that provide emotional resonance) before reverberating with certain physical cells in our internal ear. Again, each cell resonates only with those vibrations that it is attuned to. This resonance symbolically reflects back our own mental and emotional flow. Through hearing we perceive an emotional and mental reflection of our spiritual self. Hearing is also a feedback mechanism mirroring our beliefs according to our spiritual path. And, again, we sometimes reject the feedback and become hard (emotionally stationary) of hearing.

Light, sound and all other vibrations are oscillations (dynamic polarities) that disturb the status quo of universal oneness. These polarities make it possible for us to experience life through the senses (**Figure 12**). Vibrations always oscillate between two complimentary polarities. All that is life and all that

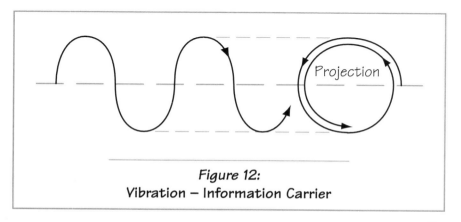

Figure 12:
Vibration – Information Carrier

is not life is in fact a vast ocean of vibrations, pulsating at different rates. All vibrations, all life, come from the original oneness (symbol of God) as a point of equilibrium and will return to oneness, thus closing the circle of life.

Part V

THE SYMBOLIC MESSAGE OF ILLNESS

❖ ❖ ❖

*"It is a mirror, but they don't always know that.
If they recognize that they've created it,
then they can change it."*

❖ ❖ ❖

Overview

From this point forward, each section describing one specific illness will be accompanied by an example. The example will be a short story that better illustrates the general aspects of that illness. Even though short, these examples, together with the general part, are the result of hours and hours of research, study and meditation. The symbolic implications and connections may not be obvious in every case.

For the purpose of describing typical cases of one illness and one illness only, and in order to avoid the confusion that may occur from talking about many clustered conditions that occur together and interrelate, (as in many real life cases), I carefully constructed each case. In all examples I selected the typical symptoms of that illness together with their explanation, and constructed a case around them. Real life cases would not be appropriate in this book because they would complicate issues and would introduce hidden connections with other emotional states in every case, thus making it nontypical.

Since all of these examples are a deviation from healthy life, they may at times seem negative to you even though they are not intended to be so. Try and take a step beyond the negative connotation of a word when you think you find one, and remind yourself that these diseases are *abnormal* patterns.

I suggest that we first perceive the denial and then be open to implementing a change. If I told you the positive aspects and then told you that you need to change, you would not know why. You would bypass the denial – the negative part – and this would not be a complete process. Furthermore, the essence of every particular illness IS this denial; and what may emerge from this denial are more or less unique, positive improvements. These personal, unique steps toward improvement are difficult to take if we are not first aware of the denial process. It is essential to understand the denial process if we want to be fully aware of what is going on.

To meet the reader's need to look up various symptoms and diseases, I have included the most common ones in this book. However, it obviously would not be practical to go into tiny details or fancy illnesses. It is difficult to give quick answers to the most commonly asked questions, such as: "But what is the meaning of this specific symptom or that specific illness?" Individual symptoms need to be analyzed one by one for symbolic patterns, and then the patterns need to be integrated with the overall situation. Sometimes the connections are strikingly obvious, but many times we need to go beyond appearances and find a new way of seeing those connections. The whole process is by no means a "shot from the hip." I believe it is more appropriate at this stage to see the whole picture.

The made-up examples in this book are to help you more fully understand the whole process. The symbolic explanations are by no means exclusive or absolute. Please do not force yourself to accept something that is not valid for yourself. Sometimes your logic may tell you something, but your intuition something else. I suggest you follow your intuition.

OSTEOARTHRITIS

Talking about osteoarthritis means talking about the most common joint disease of human beings. It also means talking about flexibility versus rigidity, stability versus stubbornness. What we call osteoarthritis is a symbolic process, slowly taking place in the joints of the elderly. The site of the affected joints varies according to the symbolic significance of a person's emotional and mental thought patterns.

A joint consists of two bone ends (dense physical support structures) separated by one or two sheets of cartilage (smooth weight bearing surfaces that glide effortlessly over each other). This physical structure is surrounded by a fibrous capsule that defines the physical boundaries of movement. The capsule is filled with synovial fluid, representative of the emotional involvements necessary in order to carry out the symbolical movements.

Movements occur within the boundaries defined by the fibrous capsule (physical limits of symbolic movement). The shape and integrity of the cartilage and bone (the belief structure and expectations) also define the physical limits of symbolic movements.

The physical world presents us with many unpredictable situations that require creativity, spontaneity, adaptability and courage. This provides us with a sense of freedom and accomplishment. If every situation was to be approached in the same predictable manner, there would be no room for fun or excitement. In other words, life as we know it would not exist without flexibility.

Joints are symbolic of this flexibility. All choices and movements are made in alignment with several axes or, symbolically speaking, in alignment with higher guidance. Joints register our degree of receptivity toward life experiences and opportunities. They are sensitive instruments indicating the current level of freedom that we allow ourselves to experience. As we get older, there is a tendency to adopt more rigid rules of living. More events are perceived to fall outside our set opinions of what is acceptable and what is not. Any new or unusual turn of events that goes against the norm is rejected or criticized. We cling to the accepted norm as a reference, even though it may have slightly slipped out of our own axis (see **Figure 13**).

Criticism shows a lack of approval of anything beyond our accepted norm. There is always a lack of approval for new, unusual directions in life when we criticize. The old, accepted norm is seen as the way to go, even though it may stifle our spontaneous desire. A right axis, symbolic of our spontaneous desire, is represented by an optimum angle at which a joint is supposed to function. In other words, seeing wrong is a mirror of a new right and wrong axis that slips into a new position. The two bones that form the joint slide a little bit from the normal and optimal angle into a new position which symbolically represent a new axis of reference for the concepts of right and wrong.

Joints symbolically define our ability to bend with physical structures and adapt to different rules. The more we accept change, the more flexible our joints will be. Symbolically, we may slide, rotate or twist rules and events forwards and backwards with different degrees of fluidity.

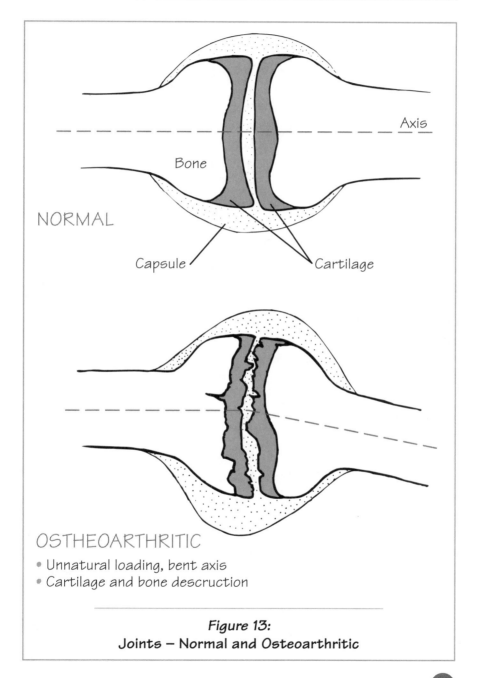

Figure 13:
Joints – Normal and Osteoarthritic

In osteoarthritis we lean toward rigid rules of living that make us carry an unnatural load. Muscles pull in unnatural directions and tighten in difficult positions.

Arthritics play the part of the silent victim. They complain very little and are generally very patient. This is why osteoarthritic lesions contain almost no inflammatory changes. These individuals never exhibit angry, violent or rebellious behavior, but rather are characterized by a stoic resistance, in spite of overbearing difficulties. They tend to be busy people that work for others and don't allow themselves to be free. The more restricted this expression of freedom, the more restrictive the range of motion in the joint.

Different joints have different degrees of freedom, depending upon the specific emotional energies that are processed by the various points in the body. For example, the range of motion of the shoulder (which has a processing function) is wider than that of the ankle (which has an elimination function). For a detailed illustration of this energy flow through the body please refer back to **Figure 5** (page 70).

In osteoarthritis, there is a change in the cartilage, the physical support structure upon which the bones glide smoothly. Enzymes, which are symbolic catalysts for change, disrupt the physical structure of cartilage fibers and allow more fluids (more emotions) to enter into the cartilage.

Symbolically, a person's movements are then based less on physical realities and more on emotional attitudes. There will be a new sense of morality that leads to rigid discipline of emotions. Then, in this patient's opinion, action in response to emotions should be controlled and limited, and emotions themselves should be (symbolically) disciplined. Consequently, more fluids (emotions) enter the cartilage and bones to create small lakes and cysts, symbolic of trapped emotions that are not allowed to flow. The water content (the emotional charge) of the cartilage increases, thus making the joint more vulnerable to physical damage from bone movement.

Eventually, this damage leads to changes in bone structure, such as minor fractures (feeling lack of support), cysts and bone reactions. Further limitations of the range of motion are imposed by new bone growth around the joint and fibrosis of the capsule, called calcifications and osteophytes. Marginal bone overgrowth symbolically reflects further physical restriction of choices. Concepts and ideas will manifest in rigid physical experiences that block the freedom of movement and, when taken to an extreme, may block the joint completely; this is called ankylosis.

Pain and stiffness are the two major complications of osteoarthritis. At first, these symptoms occur after a period of rest or immobility and are transitory. They are felt during the initial phases of movement, as if the joint needed time to decide whether or not to participate in certain situations. Stiffness is a symbolic reflection of a rigid philosophy, an increase in consistency and lack of adaptative flexibility. By limiting movement and change, stiffness limits the expression of life itself. Denial of certain aspects of oneself is painful. Joint pain (discussed in greater detail on pages 78 through 80) has to do with denial of the unnatural burden on the joint and refusal to adapt to new situations. When the condition is allowed to progress, the symptoms become more or less permanent. This denial of active participation in spite of the inner desire to do so, creates an emotional pressure felt as pain. Pain usually helps us remember that something is not flowing naturally on the physical, emotional, mental or spiritual levels.

Osteoarthritis Example: Ethel

Ethel is a 55-year-old working mother of three children. She is overly active and does home chores and work assignments remarkably well. She likes to tell everybody what to do and often believes she is the only one who can accomplish what needs to be done. Ethel tends to feel limited because of her unique qualities that force her to benevolently take charge. She never complains or gets angry because she has learned to control her emotions. She deeply believes she is a good example of the way society should be.

Yet she has the nagging feeling that over time this life of routine, hard work and self sacrifice will bring her to a dead end. It has been a long time since she allowed anything really new or fascinating in her lifestyle.

One morning after a busy work week, Ethel wakes up feeling stiffness in the left hip. Symbolically, her ability to freely accept a wide range of expression is reduced and needs to be acknowledged. When she tries to step forward she feels pain. Pain here is an expression of a subconscious denial of different experiences. That denial is initially directed toward her unusually heavy work load at home and at her job.

Ethel has difficulties accepting the self-imposed limits of freedom. Exercising her freedom to move forward makes her feel better and the pain lessens after several minutes of walking. This is typical in osteoarthritis. But the message of pain still needs to be accessed. When she goes to sleep, she has a dream about being on an endless road through a desert, while more adventurous side paths are tempting her to green oases. Ethel wakes up and remembers her dream, then thinks, "Forget it, I have a lot of things to do; let's get ready for work." She moves to get up, and at this precise moment a wave of intense pain shoots through her hip again. She continues to limp all day. Walking on her usual path is now painful because she is rejecting her intuitions, instead of following them.

Days pass by. At the start of each new day (or new movement), pain is a reminder of her need to allow herself more freedom and be less judgmental of others. At times, when she is caring more for herself and being less judgmental of others, the pain lessens. If she persists in her way of being, her condition will become chronic and her hip will eventually be painful even at rest. Symbolically, this means that to remain in her present situation is painful to her.

However, her conditioning of what a good mother and wife is supposed to be, might tempt her to stay in the present rut. What she needs to acknowledge now is to be spontaneous and enjoy her natural way of being, without criticism or judgment.

HEADACHES AND MIGRAINES

Migraines and headaches are some of the most frequent human discomforts. Symbolic analysis proves useful in helping us gain an understanding of this ailment. Let us begin by breaking the word headache into its components: head and ache. The head is the center of the intellect, will power and wisdom. The head represents conscious and subconscious thoughts and is symbolically in charge of the whole body.

Ache or pain is an overwhelming subject in medical literature. Massive volumes have been filled with research on pain. But although certain pain substances and pain fibers have been discovered and documented, their mechanisms are as yet poorly understood. Because of the vast range of subjective variability of pain, its real nature escapes scientific approach. Throughout human history, the sensation of pain has been associated with many subconscious processes. The closest origin of the word pain has to do with punishment and, therefore, with a sense of guilt. Since ancient times, mankind has believed that pain and suffering were inflicted by God. People's acts were supposed to be rewarded if they were good; but condemned and punished if bad. One might say that the ancient Gods were mirroring the ways and ideas of their ancient society. Gods were made to be cruel because people were thinking in terms of cruelty. It is important to realize that all judgment is ultimately a mirror of self-judgment.

These ideas about judgment and punishment are a legacy deeply engraved in the subconscious minds of modern mankind. Quick to judge and label, modern man functions in ways quite similar to his ancestor. The reward/punishment system is still in place, albeit more subtle and buried deeper in the subconscious. You may believe that if you follow a bad diet, you will have stomach pains, or that if you smoke, you will be punished with lung cancer. Things are not necessarily so, but if you believe them to be so, you will find them to be true for yourself. Punishment is a creation of individual and collective subconscious beliefs.

Let's say, for example, that a person (we'll name him "Tom") mishandles a situation to a point where a good friend is fired from his/her job. Tom may feel guilty and believe that he deserves punishment. A few days later, he may be the victim of an automobile accident where his arm is broken and his head bruised. This will create long-standing pain which, in his belief system, is well deserved, because his pain fulfills a need in this reward/punishment system. The degree of pain and injury will be in direct relationship to the degree of his guilt.

The idea of punishment invokes an external force and implies a dualistic world view of good/bad, or perpetrator/victim, etc. Let's try to rise above these polarizing aspects in order to understand pain from a new, neutral perspective. The practice of labeling situations in terms of good and bad is subjective by its very nature and implies splitting unity into opposites. In our example, Tom could just as well be convinced that the firing of his friend is a good thing, thereby triggering a rewarding chain of events, like him being promoted and the friend finding a much better position. There is always the option of considering the other side of the coin. Being able to see both sides of a situation without taking sides is an art that leads to more complete and truthful understanding. And, once we get beyond the temptation of labeling actions or beliefs as good or bad, the need for subconscious punishment will disappear!

This book is based on a simple optimistic premise: every symptom, every disease, everything bad exists to help us in some way. Diseases and difficulties are in fact custom-made symbolic messages designed to assist us in finding our path. All we have to do is decode these messages and give the guidance permission to take place.

So, how can pain be helpful with anything? The answer is that pain is a cry for recognition. It signals that some area in our life is in need of attention. Once attention is given and the issue resolved, the pain subsides. Example: place your hand in a fire and you will most likely experience intense pain. If you withdraw your hand quickly enough, the pain will disappear. If you deny the issue and stay in the fire, the pain will intensify. The more the pain is denied, the more it increases, in order to avoid irreversible damage or death (of the hand). Once the hand dies, the message is outdated and you no longer feel pain.

Pain, therefore, signals that something has deviated from the most beneficial flow of life and, if allowed to continue, will produce symbolic death. When we don't make appropriate changes, we act in disharmony with our purpose. Some might call this type of action wrong-doing and experience guilt. Punishment, in their minds, follows as a natural consequence. In fact, people create punishment in their lives according to their beliefs. For example, let's say someone subconsciously believes that sexual promiscuity is a bad thing that deserves punishment. After participating in such activity, this person could attract venereal disease and pain – which is then perceived as an inevitable consequence.

Pain is always associated with denial, which causes the stream of life energy to be blocked. On the physical level, this usually manifests as a diminished blood supply (symbolic of emotions) to the affected area.

Resistance to the flow of inner feelings creates suffering, confusion and control issues. We want life to flow in safe channels, even though this may not be what we really need deep inside. In such situations we find ourselves mentally forcing the life patterns into the well-known rut while tossing away opportunities for unique, new patterns that yearn for recognition.

For example, David under social pressure may want to become a doctor or a lawyer ignoring an inner calling to be free and travel around the world. This denial may cause mental, emotional and finally physical pain in body areas symbolically related to the issue. The purpose of the pain is to grab David's attention so that he will recognize the inner need and act upon it. As a doctor or lawyer, David will be faced with more emotional and mental strains than his colleagues. His belief in guilt, punishment, suffering and pain will eventually come true. David will be more prone to physical and mental illnesses. As a doctor, his patients will mirror his pain and suffering at different levels; as a lawyer, his clients will mirror his confusion. Lawyers and doctors are susceptible to physical illnesses – not because of their clients, who are just innocent mirrors, but because of their own internal processes.

There is always a close symbolic connection between the type of denial and the character of the pain, whether it be acute or chronic, sharp or dull, pressure-like or staggering. Headaches represent mental energies (thoughts) not in alignment with inner wisdom.

Different areas of the brain have different symbolic functions. The anterior (front) side relates to the future; the post-centralis area (brain midline) represents the present moment; while the posterior (back) side relates to the past (please refer to **Figure 14**). This midline is a well known anatomical reference. More specifically, the pre-frontal area (which literally means in front of your forehead) deals with forethought and planning. The way we choose to act is governed by the area immediately in front of (anterior to) the midline. Our feelings that respond to what happened a moment ago are projected just posterior to (behind) the midline (see **Figure 15**).

The symbolic significance of vision serves as an excellent example. In order for us to physically see an object, the object needs to be in a physical form. The physical form is the product of long-standing beliefs, emotions and mental processes. It takes time for these mental and emotional processes to manifest as

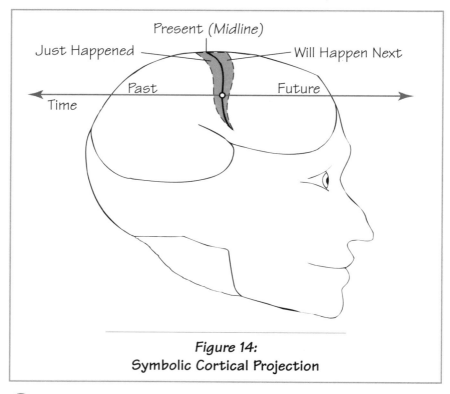

Figure 14:
Symbolic Cortical Projection

actual physical forms. Let us say we decide to build a house. From the moment we first imagine the house to the moment the house is built, a period of time passes. When we later see this house, it is the result of wishes and mental processes from the past. Accordingly, the vision center is symbolically located in the far back of the brain. Sound vibrations are a reflection of more recent emotional events, which is why they are processed closer to the midline.

The side of the head that is involved in a headache is also revealing much about its symbolic meaning. Ancient Chinese philosophy has long postulated what modern science is now redis-covering: the flow of the universe is based upon an internal inter-play of opposite forces. The complementary pairs of Yin and

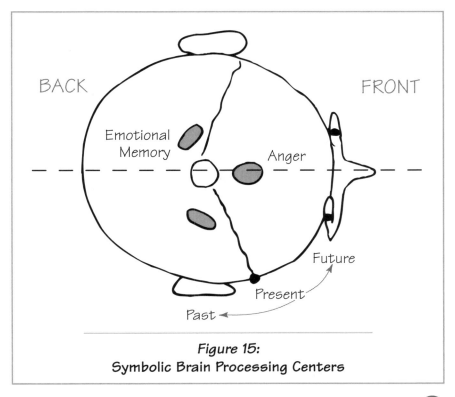

Figure 15:
Symbolic Brain Processing Centers

Yang, light and dark, masculine and feminine, etc., come together to create the world as we know it. These forces are like two sides of a coin that define and complete each other. One cannot exist without the other. It comes as no surprise that the left brain hemisphere controls the right side of the body and vice versa. There are fibers that cross in the midline for a short symbolic midline contact with each other, the contact point representing balance and unity. This phenomenon of crossing sides at the midline indicates that there exists mutual regulation among the two qualities. In other words, left balances right and right balances left. For an easier understanding, please see **Figure 16**.

The right brain/left side of the body corresponds to the feminine aspects of nature which include Yin qualities such as creativity, intuition, receptivity, introversion, and being responsive to life experiences. They symbolize our feminine qualities (every human being has both masculine and feminine qualities), which are reflected back to us through our mothers, wives, daughters, and other females in our surroundings.

The left brain/right side of the body relates to the masculine energies, which include Yang qualities such as logic, action, extroversion, giving, forward orientation and constructing life experiences. They symbolize our masculine qualities which are reflected back to us through husbands, fathers, sons, and all other males.

In light of what we just discussed, headaches have a distinct symbolic significance that deals with control issues and a refusal to see the bigger picture of a situation. Headaches signify an attempt to escape realities, be they physical, mental, emotional or spiritual. The three major benign type of headaches are illustrated in and **Table 7** and **Figure 17**:

1) Pain on one side: *Migraine headache;*
2) Diffuse pain: *Tension headache;* and
3) Pain above the eye while sleeping: *Cluster headache.*

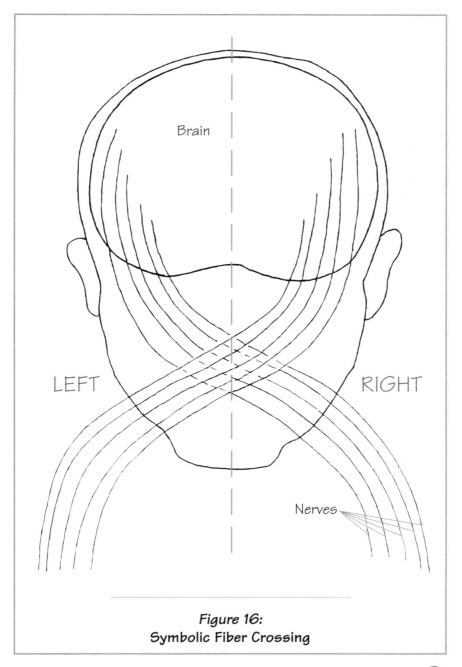

Figure 16:
Symbolic Fiber Crossing

Table 7: Characteristics of Headaches		
MIGRAINE:	TENSION:	CLUSTER:
One-sided	Top of head	Above the eye
Intense	Pressure like	Extremely intense
Premonitory symptoms	Diffuse or bandlike	Nightly for weeks, while dreaming
Aggravated by many factors	During intense stress	Craving for air, suicide risk
Prevalent in females	Depression danger	Prevalent in males

Classic Migraine

A classic migraine is a one-sided headache common in young women. It occurs every few weeks, usually in the mornings, and is sometimes preceded by premonitory visual or auditory symptoms (the patient can tell that the headache is about to hit). Symbolically, migraine is a denial of one aspect of the personality, generally the left hemisphere (the masculine, logical side), although it may very well be the right, feminine side. A left brain denial (remember that the brain symbolism switches sides) may indicate a denial of active assertiveness in social settings or interpersonal relationships.

Left brain denial may be triggered by situations that directly evoke the troubled issue, or by symbolic representations such as: consumption of red wine or other alcoholic beverages (they cause one to drop inhibitions and mind games); lights (symbolic of the light of our path or of seeing points of view in different lights); chocolate (sex related issues); coffee and tea (sweet emotional excitement); premenstrual tensions (heightened feminine issues).

Migraine usually strikes in the morning when we begin a new day, a new life project. The affected person cannot tolerate light (symbolic of the higher light of a situation, the light at the end of a tunnel or simply the truth), or sounds (higher emotional messages or warnings). In extreme cases, the refusal to act on or

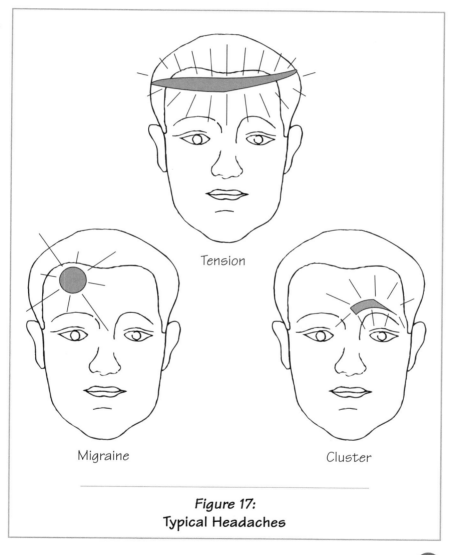

Tension

Migraine

Cluster

Figure 17:
Typical Headaches

see a particular aspect of life leads literally to paralysis or partial blindness.

During the entire migraine attack, there is diminished blood flow to various areas of the brain and diminished vascular response, both of which are indicative of denial of spiritual guidance. This type of pain may linger for the whole day, but usually subsides at night when the logical side goes to sleep.

MIGRAINE EXAMPLE: TRACY

Tracy is a 22-year-old college student with an active lifestyle, who has many friends and a loving family. She enjoys life and is used to having lots of fun. Her boyfriend is supportive. Days and nights were just not long enough for Tracy.

Semester finals were approaching. They were a bit challenging, so Tracy thought she would start studying Monday. Meanwhile, she would enjoy the weekend, go to a party, have fun and relax.

Monday morning, after a cup of coffee, Tracy felt strange. Letters and small lights were dancing in front of her eyes, and for the first time in her life, she couldn't concentrate.

Tracy knew she needed to refocus her life around studying, at least for a period of time. But while she was focusing on the exam materials, she suddenly had a headache on the left side, just above her left temple. (Symbolically, this meant that she denied the logical, controlling part of her that was forcing her to study.) She couldn't concentrate on the textbook.

Tracy went to a dark room (subconscious refuge; refusal to see the light of the situation). The touch of objects and the sound of noise affected her strongly (she didn't want to be reminded of the present circumstances). She resented the pressure of her deadlines and felt nauseated. It was all a symbolic temper tantrum. Gone were the exciting times of no worries. Coffee and a box of chocolate (symbolic substitutes for excitement) worsened the pain instead of sweetening it. Even trying to think logically was painful.

Tracy recognized that studying took more determination and will power than she was accustomed to. She made a conscious decision that she did want to take these exams and succeed.

After getting used to the idea of concentrated studying, the pain became more bearable. Over the next several days, Tracy noticed that routine helped her overcome her resistance. She wasn't fighting or denying anymore, and her pain subsided. She did pass her examinations successfully.

Tracy had entered a more self-controlled phase of her life. Nevertheless, she still sometimes subconsciously rejected major tasks that seemed challenging or time consuming. During these times, she had headaches and craved the spice of life, symbolized by sweets, tea, coffee, chocolate or red wine. She came to believe that these food indulgences were to blame for her migraines, not realizing that they were only symbolic associations.

At 36, Tracy was married with two children and had a good job. Her work load was reasonable and provided her with a balanced mixture of routine and fun. She was still having migraines from time to time.

One Saturday morning, when she had planned a big spring cleaning, she woke up with her left-sided migraine. The pain stayed there that whole weekend. But, surprisingly, Monday morning the pain was gone.

Next weekend Tracy decided to hire somebody for the cleaning job and she went out and had fun. Without consciously realizing it, she just avoided another migraine attack.

Tension Headaches

Tension related headaches are a diffuse, pressure-like pain that is felt across the top of the head or as a band-like throbbing. These types of headaches are common in middle-aged individuals and occur during intense moments of emotional stress, worry or depression. They continue for weeks or months and are hardly affected by painkillers. Depression will be discussed later in greater detail; suffice it to say that its symbolic association has to do with victimhood and the avoidance of inspirational desires and dreams that we need in order to advance on our unique path. During a period of crisis, a middle-aged individual may insist on clinging to his/her familiar rut out of social pressure, lack of self-confidence, or simply out of inertia. Depression means doubting our personal power to create reality.

The top of the head is an energetic vortex, symbolic of cosmic unity and greater understanding of life and the circle is a symbol of unmanifest unity pulsating in harmony with the rhythm of nature. A painful pulsating circle on top of the head is designed to remind us of our ultimate path toward the blissful union with the forces of the universe. The inner beckoning to one's spiritual bliss is suppressed and manifests as a circular pressure on the top of the head. Tension headache indicates that a person is at a spiritual crossroads, and will remain as long as this issue is not acknowledged.

Cluster Headaches

Cluster headache is an extremely intense, short, constant one-sided pain above the eye, usually occurring in males during dreaming (not merely sleeping). It is associated with eye symptoms on the same side and may recur nightly for weeks or months (clusters), especially during emotionally upsetting experiences. Pain above the affected eye is accompanied by closure of the eyelid and the pupil, all of which suggests a refusal to see an issue. The patient is gasping for air (oxygen, the spiritual life force, is needed). Sometimes the pain becomes so intense that it can lead to suicide.

While dreaming, we connect to a level of consciousness that cannot be understood in the waking state. Dreams provide access to the guidance of our higher consciousness, where we can resolve issues that may be difficult to handle in the limited world of physical existence. The spiritual guidance of dreams is so essential to life that we cannot survive without it any more than we could survive without oxygen (symbolic of spiritual energy). Experiments have shown that animals who were allowed to sleep, but were awakened when they began to dream, started exhibiting unusual, dysfunctional behaviors and eventually died or even killed themselves.

The intense sensation of pain at the beginning of a dream is related to an intense denial of a crucial aspect of our spiritual path. Subconsciously, an agreement has been made, but the individual is refusing to carry it out. When he is reminded of his calling during the dream, the patient responds with an intense denial and refusal to see. Once the guidance is finally accepted, the pain resolves. This type of headache generally affects men, probably because they tend to be more reluctant to accept guidance.

BACK PAINS, SPRAINS AND ACCIDENTS

Since pain has already been discussed in the chapter on Headaches and Migraines, let us now examine the symbolic significance of bone structures. Bones are hard and compact compared to body fluids and tissues, as they represent the density of our inner structure and support. They are the slowest to change, and when they do change, this generally requires a profound process that involves all the layers of manifestation – from the spiritual, mental and emotional all the way to the physical ("down to the bone").

Symbolically, all the bones are constructed out of three basic geometric shapes: the circle, triangle and square (see **Figure 18**). It is as if they borrowed symbolic attributes from geometry – their energy flows easily from the unmanifested unity and unbounded freedom of the circle through the creative energy of the triangle to the materialization of the square.

The triangle, the creative symbol and origin of all forms, is the simplest geometric shape representative of the transition between transcendental and material. Mathematics has its basis in the triangle, as does geometry. The triangle symbolizes a

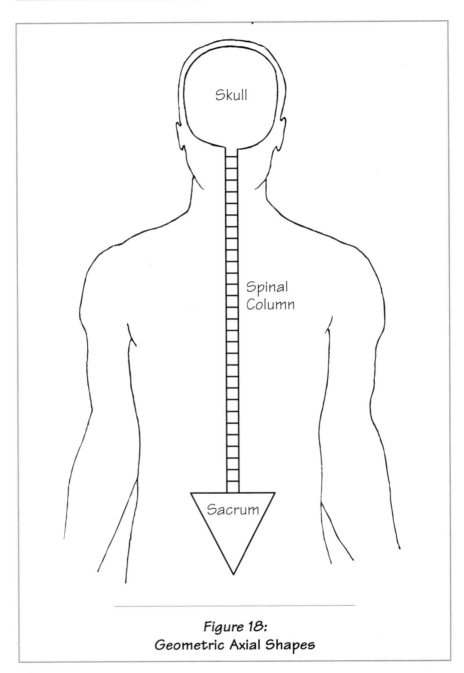

Figure 18:
Geometric Axial Shapes

sacred, creative transition from pure mathematical potentiality to manifest physical reality.

All human vertebrae contain a series of balanced circles, triangles and squares. In the human skeleton, round shapes are generally placed in axial locations, while long bones are found peripherally. This pattern of spreading outward from a core follows nature's basic law of manifestation and can be observed in many creatures and natural formations. The sacrum denotes the sacred triangle, "mother of form." It has symbolic implications in anchoring the physicality and, not coincidentally, shaping the birth canal, the passage we all emerge from when we take on a physical form (see **Figure 19**).

Both the sacrum and the coccyx consist of five vertebrae that are fused together. Ten (two pairs of five) is the symbol of infinite potential manifesting as divine individuality. Five is the number of life, comprised of three plus two (three stands for the masculine, two stands for the feminine). The human spinal column contains five lumbar vertebrae that are symbolically related to the physical realities (the five senses). Above these are the twelve emotion-related vertebrae (twelve is the number of completion), and seven cervical, mental vertebrae (seven is the number of wisdom). Note that all these numbers are combinations of five and seven. The seven cervical (mental) and five lumbar (physical) vertebrae add up to a complete twelve once again.

Lower back pain or tension is a familiar discomfort to most of us because pain or denial at the level of these structures is frequent. Back pain is a leading cause of disability in people less than forty-five years of age, an overwhelming number of them being males. Bones symbolize physical support, emotional strength and stability, and they also represent our personal spiritual support structures materialized in the physical realm.

Burdens of physical and material responsibility, as well as lack of financial backing, show in the lower back.

Mental rigidity affects the cervical area. In osteoarthritis there is a classic weakness at the C6-C7 level, signifying a rough relationship between these two vertebrae in the neck. Symbolically, this indicates a discordance between C6 (the ability to praise and give thanks) and C7 (the faculty of rational thinking).

A vast majority of adult males experience problems at the juncture between S_1 and L_5, where the spine meets the sacrum.

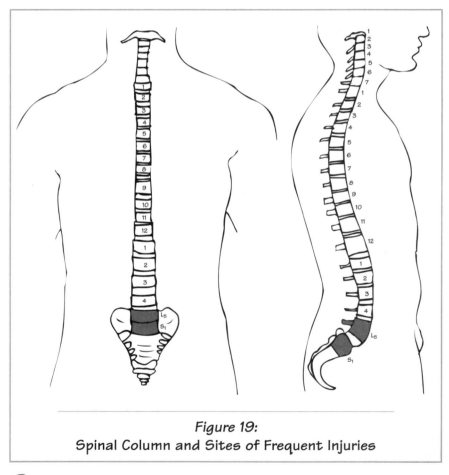

Figure 19:
Spinal Column and Sites of Frequent Injuries

Symbolically speaking, they have difficulties accepting the sacredness of material existence and tend to deny or distrust the sacred spiritual support of physical materiality. It is typical for the average Western, money-oriented individual to be consumed with financial worries and doubt his capacity to financially materialize support (through spiritual experience).

Many people resent monthly bills and distrust their ability to pay them. When this confidence and trust is shaken, back pain is a common occurrence. It is interesting to note that in Third World countries, where people more readily trust that nature will provide for tomorrow's needs, back pain is not a common occurrence, even though they may perform harder physical labor. Generally, back pain is more frequent in males, and is especially predominant in individuals and societies that believe in hard work as the only way to survive.

Lower back pain almost always involves issues of control over some particular pathways. There pathways are physical, but close to the sacrum – the sacred spiritual support of the spinal column, therefore they are usually related to our ability to manifest financial support.

The nerves of the back are the physical mirror of the paths we choose in life. When a disc slips, it presses upon a nerve and causes pain. In the language of symbolism, we can say that the restraints of unfavorable circumstances (such as a tight budget) are usually perceived as external pressure beyond our control. Our control of the situation is threatening to slip away; symbolically we experience this as pressure or as a pinch. This pressure may be symbolically correlated with a slipped disc and pinched nerve. A shooting pain down to the feet may follow during this situation, with its corresponding symbolic significance – a sharp denial of justice and goodness in the universe.

Sprains, Fractures and Accidents

At this point it is probably clear to you that, symbolically speaking, all accidents are a build-up of internal pressures that suddenly burst into the physical realm and disrupt its status quo. Strong deviations from genuine personal journeys and rebellion against physical realities attract accidents. Rebellious teenagers are especially prone to them, as your local insurance statistics can confirm.

All events, good or bad, serve as messages of love and as reminders of new perspectives. Sometimes they help us break boundaries that no longer serve us. By consciously recognizing the degree of rebellion building up inside and by acknowledging the emotional and mental messages, it is possible to resolve these disruptions without the need to experience them physically. Accidents are avoidable, unless we need them in a deeper spiritual way. Sprains are the consequence of movements beyond the normal range. Outrageous thought patterns that interfere with one's plans can physically manifest as sprains, usually at the ankles. The ankle is the place of integration between the vertical and horizontal planes; they signify a symbolic crossing that gives birth to our path and direction to our steps. Therefore, clutching to old plans that are not aligned with our current needs can translate into repetitive ankle sprains.

Fractures denote the symbolic breaking of a support system or rigid psychological system. The external forces that cause the break are an expression of internal conflicts (mental or emotional) that shatter the trust in an established physical reality. Additional clues about the symbolic cause of a fracture can be derived from the exact location of the break. A fracture may involve a joint, indicating issues around flexibility and freedom of movement; or it may affect a long bone, denoting conflicts with physical rules that have long been established. If the symbolic cause of the trauma is severe, the fracture can penetrate through the skin or dislocate bones from a joint. In these cases, the accumulated tension has disrupted an inflexible, unyielding system to the point where parts of the physical reality are not even contained within emotional limits, which are symbolically indicated by the fluid in the joint capsule.

A fracture is a physical bone destruction symbolizing a sudden loss of sustenance (a fractured bone cannot sustain us), which originates from thought patterns that do not sustain us. When this happens, the overall harmony of the mental-emotional-physical unit suffers a literal crash. Internal lesions and hemorrhage restrict normal blood supply (spiritual energy and information) only to that specific area, which further impairs the range of motion.

Accidents are a symbolic mirror of our problems. Did we forget to slow at the yield sign, or did we just not see the other car? Were we symbolically looking in the wrong direction? Did we (symbolically) fall asleep, or are we having trouble with our passing maneuvers?

Accidents may reveal to us a missed opportunity to change course in life. The lack of conscious courage to abandon an old path can lead us to a symbolic head-on collision.

BACK PAIN EXAMPLE: ALEX

Our subject for back pain will be Alex, a 36-year-old, otherwise healthy individual. He was raised to believe that only hard work can bring him success, and always worked in one way or another since the age of sixteen.

Even though deep inside he feels the connection with the sacred part of existence, he doesn't pay too much attention to it in every day living. His parents are somewhat religiously inclined, but Alex grew up believing more in himself than in outside help. His sense of orderliness and organization have served to fuel his self-confidence and a desire for greater accomplishments.

During his college days he experienced back pain for the first time – while studying for an examination, although his mind was on financial pressures. He needed money for a vacation and a new car. Up until then he had relied on his parents for extra cash, but they were ill and he had to take care of them.

Suddenly, Alex's self confidence was challenged. He felt forced to get an extra job because his part-time delivery job wasn't providing enough. He didn't feel supported. Weeks passed, he felt tired and overworked and his confidence took a nose dive.

He was on his own and his schedule was getting busier and busier. One day while delivering a large package and thinking about the challenges of making money on his own he experienced pain on the right side of his back for the first time. Before this thought was even finished, a sudden pain shot through his lower back. He stopped, held his breath (didn't want to accept it) and put the package down. The pain subsided a little.

Alex took off from work that day, but the pain continued to persist, especially when stretching or while doing rotatory movements. Alex was being challenged in his belief that hard work is the only way to provide.

Alex needed to acknowledge his subconscious choice for this challenge. He needed to look at this situation with trust and acceptance. He needed to acknowledge a sacred support to the logical, constructive way he wanted to manifest the financial supply. By not acknowledging nature's ability to provide financial support, he considered himself without spiritual support. Pain came when he was overworked, mirroring the general overload in his life.

But what exactly was happening? The smooth connection between the sacred and the physical – the S_1/L_5 discs – had become distorted and was pinching the nerve connection to the leg. Symbolically, this meant that he was feeling external pressure on his own logical control mechanisms (nerves that govern his path and way of being). Just as Alex felt he was slipping away from his support system, his disc slipped in his lower back.

Alex did manage to get through those difficult days, graduated from college and improved his financial situation, but he could never forget them. He didn't completely understand what happened and did not quite learn the trust lesson he was supposed to have learned. For this reason, his back pains continued several times a year, usually during times of financial distress.

Later, he married and continued to work overtime to pay a mortgage. By the time his first child was born, Alex felt burdened by responsibilities and his back pains returned more strongly. His pain usually set in late in the afternoon, when he was overworked or when missing his family: Nourishment is a symbolic form of support, therefore he was also in pain when missing the emotional nourishment that his family provides.

His pains intensified when trying to stretch or bend (see the symbolism here). However, Alex didn't end up with permanent back pain. As soon as his wife started to work again, he felt better, and after obtaining a bank loan the pain disappeared.

Family life is helping to change Alex's philosophy about material possessions; now he is discovering that he worries less about money and enjoys more of his life. His pain was his friend, and Alex subconsciously acknowledged the message, even though consciously he was not aware of it. Intuition led him to a healthier lifestyle and more fulfilling experiences.

HIGH BLOOD PRESSURE

High blood pressure and heart attacks, hotly debated topics nowadays, have been briefly surveyed in this book. Without losing ourselves in millions of technical details, we need to comprehend the symbolic implications of major disease processes. Through careful study of these health conditions, we realize how little is understood about them. Research and theories abound, but the answers to our essential questions, "Why me, why now, and why these symptoms and not something else?" are far from being addressed. When we find massive research projects on a particular subject, this tends to point out just how little is known about that subject, since research is generally not done on things that are considered known and self-evident.

Individuality becomes lost in statistics. For example, if you have a 50% chance of survival in a year, this is just a fancy scientific way of saying, "Maybe you'll die, maybe not, we don't know." It is important to realize that this chance of survival exists only for an outside observer, not for you. At the end of the year, you will either be alive or dead, not 50% of each. If you believe in a statistic which indicates that you're likely to die, then this experience will be borne out for you. However, there is no law stating that you have to behave statistically. You don't have to behave like anyone before you. You can change things if you want to; all you need is the awareness that change is required. Unique personal options are ignored in statistics. People want and need to be treated as unique personalities, because each one of us is unique and special. The personalized approach is what lends the human dimension of hope and optimism to the medical act.

In order to become aware of what needs to be changed, we may use the symbolic approach. The symbolic approach to understanding a medical condition is useful because it explains many conditions and correlations whose causes were previously not known. This approach also makes many correlations predictable.

The words "high blood pressure" and "hypertension" indicate a high degree of internal pressure and tension. The reasons why an individual may experience tension are countless, but there is one specific pattern that is required for any pressure to build up anywhere: failure to let go! If you let go easily, there will be no internal tension, no matter how much you take in. Imagine cooking in a pressure cooker with a closed valve – sooner or later it will explode. If you partially open the valve, there will be less pressure inside. If, however, you cook in an open pot, there is no pressure build up at all. The kidneys are like pressure valves for our body, so if they are open and function well, the water pressure cannot build up.

High blood pressure is symbolic of relatively long-standing emotional concerns (fluid relates to emotions) that want to be released. Like a high pressure system, these patients have unexpressed feelings, blocks, anger, anxieties or fears. Since it is blood that is under pressure, there is generally a restriction (internal or external) in fully expressing personal vitality and joy.

From this perspective, it is not difficult to understand why males, blacks or older people are exhibiting higher rates of high blood pressure, since it is not socially acceptable for these groups of individuals to express feelings easily. From this point of view, it becomes obvious that obese people, diabetics and patients with kidney problems (all with increased rates of high blood pressure and kidney problems) also have repressed vitality and difficulties with letting go, accepting and forgiving. Forgiving means giving one's focus forward instead of backward; releasing instead of holding back.

In an elastic system, the pressure of the blood is also measured by the amount of resistance that an expansion receives (see **Figure 20**). Pressure is defined by how much something presses against

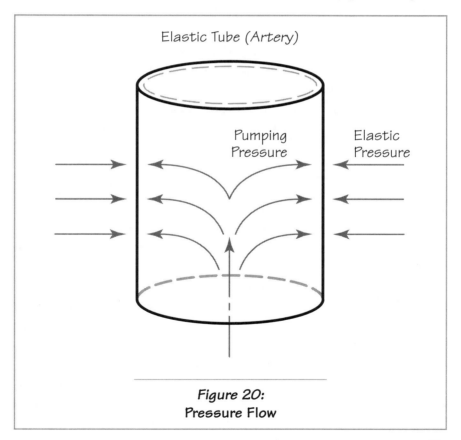

Figure 20:
Pressure Flow

something else. This measurement is expressed by two numbers: one to gauge expansion and one to keep track of resistance. In a static system with very high, nonelastic resistance (an oxygen tank for example), just one number is necessary to indicate the difference between the two forces. But in a dynamic system with wide variation in elasticity, such as the circulatory system, there is also wide variation in pressure. Numbers fluctuate between maximum and minimum expansion rates. When expansion is active, resistance becomes passive. When daylight comes, nighttime retreats. In this way, these two opposites mirror one another and define each other in a complementary fashion.

Blood pressure has two values: systolic and diastolic. The systolic (expansive) number measures how much we try to accomplish our tasks, whereas the diastolic (elastic resistance) number symbolizes what we perceive the external resistance to be. These two values come together to form a number (140/80 for example). Most of the times, these values increase or decrease simultaneously because the more stressed we are, the more resistance we perceive and, consequently, the more effort we put forth.

Research has confirmed that blood pressure increases (especially the systolic value) during outward oriented physical activities. By the same token, blood pressure decreases (especially the diastolic value) when we do inward oriented activities like meditating or sleeping.

High blood pressure can be produced by long standing tension, or it can be an acute reaction to a highly traumatic event, in which case it is called malignant. Typically, the patient is a male in his forties which is suggestive of mid-life crisis.

What each patient actually experiences differs from one individual to the other. In minor cases, there are only slight vision disturbances or occipital (back side) headaches. Occipital headaches, as discussed previously, represent denying the process of integrating what is seen. The refusal to see what is going on may physically manifest in a large spectrum of vision problems that range from small black spots to total blindness. Other typical symptoms may include:

- dizziness,
- vertigo,
- vomiting,
- paralysis,
- fainting (syncope),

- refusal to focus,
- spinning out of control,
- rejection,
- inability to move on,
- desire to escape and give up.

Long-term complications of high blood pressure are an expression of proliferation (muscular build-up) in the walls of arteries. Initial stretching of an artery occurs because of its elasticity, as a result of the increased blood pressure of the blood pulsating through. If the stretching continues for too long, a set of small muscles in the wall of the blood vessel help these vessels retain their normal shape. The more these muscles are used, the more they bulge – it's the body building concept. Symbolically, the tension is perpetuated by the physical reactions which we initiate in response to the initial tension.

These reactions provide temporary relief, but over time they become the source of more strain, which amplifies the vicious circle of tension.

For example, if we try to cover a lie with another lie, it may provide temporary relief, but in the long-term the new lie becomes a source of more strain because we need to stretch more and more to patch every possible aspect of the new lie. The tension builds up until it erupts (we get caught).

This muscular proliferation can appear anywhere in the body, but it is most intense in the eyes, kidneys and brain (it is difficult to feel in control during these times) and in the heart (which makes it hard to appreciate harmony).

Subconsciously, a patient may eventually decide to shut down the kidneys (renal failure), the heart (heart attacks and failure), the eyes (blindness) or the brain (stroke). These all indicate a symbolic need to acknowledge life processes: to love, to see, to understand and to let go.

HIGH BLOOD PRESSURE EXAMPLE: GEORGE

Let our patient be George, who was raised in a family of strict principles, obeys rules all his life and begins to adopt this lifestyle at an early age. Being in the army reinforces his tendency to follow a path dictated by others. At the same time, the army also teaches him the other side of the coin: George has a taste of independence, perseverance and success.

After his service, he gets a job, makes many friends and has a good time. Then, he marries Michelle and settles down. She was also raised in a family of rigid rules. They have children together and for some time everything seemed to be all right.

However, George still remembers the times when he was on his own. There are just too many responsibilities in his marriage. The world starts to press upon him, demanding more and more. Michelle is criticizing him frequently. Pressure is slowly building up. It is at this time in his life when his blood pressure begins to rise above normal. George doesn't feel sick and in fact has no way of knowing about his condition, because he never sees a doctor. For years, George has borderline hypertension without knowing it.

One day George has a new boss. He is more demanding, rigid in thinking and expression, and expects rules to be followed to exasperation. He assigns tasks that seem unreasonable (notice how everything mirrors his thought patterns). George initially accepts some of these tasks, but after a while they start to bother him. A new kind of pressure is building up inside him. Every little task given to George builds up his diastolic blood pressure (diastolic blood pressure symbolically corresponds to the pressure George perceives to be exerted upon him).

George begins to fight with Michelle. One day, during a minor argument, the systolic value of George's blood pressure rises proportionately higher than the diastolic one. That day, at work, he is being asked to do hard work that is not usually his responsibility. His diastolic blood pressure builds. Finally, to top it off, his new boss criticizes him heavily. George's blood pressure shoots sky high; he wants to say something, but suddenly feels dizzy and sees bright and dark spots buzzing around his head. There is a ringing in his ears. (The noise is a symbolic expression of not letting go of a specific emotional vibration.)

Alarmed by his symptoms, his colleagues accompany him to the company nurse, who finds his blood pressure to be extremely high. Symbolically, George is boiling inside like a pressure cooker. He is taken to the hospital. In the Emergency Room he is diagnosed with hypertension (high blood pressure) and admitted for observation. Far away from his problems, in the hospital, George feels better. However, he doesn't realize that when he receives flowers and well wishes from wife and boss, his blood pressure temporarily rises again.

George is finally discharged with a diagnosis of hypertension and instructions to take pills. The pills make him feel blunted and less overwhelmed, so he can return to his daily activities. These activities are not something he cannot handle, but they are far from what he would like to do. It is still not too late for

George to acknowledge his inner longings and allow more freedom into his life.

CANCER

Cancer is not an easy subject to discuss, because everyone has different opinions about this illness. There are medical societies organized around cancer, meetings about it and marches against it. Many of us will experience growths, tumors or cancers at some point in our lives, and many of us will have traumatic experiences around them. Passions are high and opinions vary.

But what is the essence and symbolic significance of this illness? As explained earlier in this book, I believe cancer, as everything in our lives, is a mirror of our consciousness. Each one of our thoughts and behaviors are reflected back to us. When we feel or behave like a cancer, we will manifest it. In the beginning, we will encounter people who display this illness as a warning. The illness will be in our minds. But it is when the issue at stake is out of control, that the cancer will start to physically take over our life.

Cancer represents different behaviors depending on type and location, but what is more important is the underlying message – the common denominator.

A tumor is a growth inside or outside the body. It grows past and beyond our organs; beyond our attitudes and belief systems. A tumor is an abnormal shape originating from an out-of-the-

154

ordinary belief system that grows out of control. Tumors take advantage of the host tissue and may cause severe damage to it. Oftentimes, when we adjust our lives according to the message the tumor symbolizes, this behavior is limited and a growth never develops into cancer. This is called a benign tumor. It is important to realize that, as in every disease, it is only when the issue is neglected and judged, that we manifest an illness. When issues are acknowledged, loved and acted upon, we usually stay healthy.

The common denominator in cancer is cell growth that has gotten out of control. These cells are mirroring deeply buried issues that want to be brought to our attention. A more profound question is: What is the behavior of a cancerous cell?

Cancerous cells do not follow the natural cycles of growth (e.g., cycles of day and night) and don't interact harmoniously with other cells. These cells lack respect, so to speak, for their neighboring cells and are out of control in both space and time. They display large amounts of energy which they steal from other cells. This is weakening and exhausting to the whole body.

Cancerous cells behave not unlike rebellious adolescents: They are independent and reluctant to take advice, break rules intentionally, and express themselves in crude, shocking ways. They have little sense of adherence to organized society (symbolized by the surrounding tissues), quickly travel to new and exciting places (metastases), and try to escape the law enforcement system (symbolized by the immune system). Cancer cells secrete enzymes that benefit their own growth while inhibiting that of their neighbors. Increased sexual activity (high index of cell divisions) is common, as are attempts to convince normal cells to follow their way. They use society as a host to be taken advantage of.

We are all familiar with this type of behavior and may occasionally catch ourselves thinking along these lines. Such thoughts can be triggered by many situations, including the

---

Table 8:
Characteristics of Cancerous Cells

Young

Independent

Strong self-expression

Growing anywhere

Out of control

Wanting fun

Lack of respect for neighboring cells

Disorganized growth

Disarrayed behavior

No sense of when to stop growing

No adherence to rules

---

stress of modern life, unresolved trauma from childhood, adolescent memories or unfulfilled desires. Each thought is followed by a corresponding emotion (energy in motion) which is reflected in the behavior of a new cell. On any given day, we probably generate many of these kind of thoughts and behaviors that make our body produce cancerous cells. If such thoughts pertain to infrequent and isolated events, so will the number and behavior of the newly formed cells: they will be smaller in number and isolated from one another. Being aware of the process always helps solve the problem faster. To use an analogy, when there is a small number of bad guys on the streets and the police are aware of them, it is relatively easy to take care of them. If, however, the bad guys are overwhelming in number, if they are organized and if they hide well, then the police are totally unaware of the problem and the situation will only get worse. Likewise, there are immune officers in charge of law and order in our body and these officers usually keep the aggressors under control.

Cancer, like everything else, is a mirror of our behavior. Perhaps cancer is becoming more and more prevalent in our society because our society is becoming more cancerous in life style and philosophy. Some qualities and behaviors displayed by the modern corporate world are astonishingly similar to those of cancer cells: The tendency to push people beyond limits, to expand and control (metastases), to subordinate the community in favor of vested interests, and to develop self-serving ideals at the expense of the community. Their ideals are placed above the interest of the collective. They overestimate their power and manipulate others in disregard for common goals.

If the experience that evoked traumatic thoughts is overpowering (like the Hiroshima bombing, for example) and has not been forgiven, then it might linger in our system. To forgive means to give for, to give attention, solve the issue and go forward. If the conflicting feelings are not expressed and resolved, they not only stay in the body, but exert pressure from the inside and rise to the surface level of conscious awareness. When they do this, we tend to again send (re-send) them back to where they came from – suppressed in the subconscious. All of a sudden we have "re-sent-ment".

If nursed long enough, these issues grow within the subconscious and will surface again and again, literally eating our life away. Cancer cells make use of some tricks to elude the immune defense mechanism, that are a reflection of the different games our subconscious thoughts play on our conscious thought patterns.

Most of the time we are unaware of our unexpressed emotions. Symbolically, a parallel can be drawn with our immune system which is unaware of cancerous cells in our system because of the tricks these cells play. In this way, cancerous cells can grow undisturbed and unacknowledged.

According to the universal mirroring concept, the organ affected by cancer symbolically represents the issue in need of more attention. We will analyze some examples of this concept here.

Leukemia is correlated with the way we defend ourselves. It is a cancer of leukocytes – a type of white blood cells which play a role in the defense mechanism of our body. If the illness is acute, there is a high degree of intensity in the response. If it is chronic, then a long, simmering process is at its basis.

After the Hiroshima bombing, there was a dramatic increase in both acute and chronic leukemias. They were all related to the *intense, acute* resentments of that specific event. The way different people *handled* those emotions determined whether the disease process was acute or chronic.

Myelogenic leukemia (originating from the granular side of white blood cells which is involved in acute reactions) is related to an acute event that we need to come to peace with, like rape or the bombing, for example.

Lymphocytic leukemia (recall that lymphocytes are involved in chronic reactions) stems from an ongoing chronic process, such as long-term abuse or oppression.

In other words, if the *cause* (the process that is perceived as difficult) is short and intense, the leukemia will be granular, whereas a long and simmering cause will result in lymphocytic leukemia.

The *individual reaction* to an event will determine whether the type of leukemia is acute or chronic. There are many combinations of all these aspects leading to a wide array of leukemia diseases with different patterns of manifestation. In essence, leukemia represents a perception of difficulty – and therefore an opportunity to move beyond our limitations.

Leukemia can occur when a person perceives him- or herself as a helpless victim of circumstances for which he or she cannot find acceptance or forgiveness. The person feels a deep resentment for their inability to defend themselves against an apparently threatening situation.

In lymphoma, the lymphatic system is affected. This system has the role of slowly carrying toxins away from the cells. If it is affected by cancer, there is a deep symbolic need to cleanse the system of emotional and mental toxins that result from long-standing hurts in life. A feeling of restriction, together with a blockage of emotional expression, are paramount in lymphoma. A typical lymphoma patient is sweet and gentle but not self-reliant, lacks motivation and relies heavily on others to get the work done. The side of the affected nodes in lymphoma indicates the location in need of attention and cleansing. If they are situated in the intestines, as in non-Hodgkin's lymphoma, the patient needs to deal with absorption and digestion of life experiences; in the neck or chest (Hodgkin's lymphoma) they signify a need for feeling, self-expression and cleansing the system; or they may be located in the brain as in AIDS, indicating a need for a mental, control-related purification.

Breast cancer has a strong correlation with a woman's sense of self. An unfulfilled desire to provide nourishment and mothering may be held inside and ultimately be expressed as breast cancer. If a woman feels she is supposed to have children and nurture them intimately, then the more she advances in life without a child, the higher her risk of developing breast cancer. The disease is prevalent in Western countries where women often delay or forego nurturing and mothering in favor of career pursuits. Life has shown that mothers who breastfeed their children for some time have a significantly reduced risk of breast cancer.

Colon cancer deals with issues of elimination. There is an unexpressed subconscious need to let go of the past, especially of material things and of outdated baggage that is not serving the person any longer. The patient would be wise to eliminate many things in order to create new spaces for new experiences.

Lung cancer reflects a latent desire for openness and receptivity to inspiration and love. This disease is a wake-up call to consciously accept love and take in new life opportunities.

Symptoms of cancer usually occur late in the course of the disease. The symptoms may be due to local effects such as invasion of local tissues or compression of the cancer onto neighboring organs, or to release of active substances into the bloodstream.

In cancer, there are different symptoms and different degrees of anger, denial, withdrawal and depression. These translate into symbolic pain, inflammatory reaction, symbolic wasting and loss of appetite. Usually, nausea and early satiety (small amount of food makes hunger disappear) indicate that food intake (intake of life experiences) is not well tolerated by these individuals.

Anemia is a frequent companion of cancer, but also of many other conditions in which less oxygen, and therefore less energy, is carried to different parts of the body. The degree of red coloration of the red blood cells (RBCs) is indicative of the intensity with which life is experienced. Red is an expression of vital force and of the fullness of an experience in the present moment. When these experiences are suppressed, denied or forgotten, we may develop anemia. Toxins, diet and other carcinogens are usually nothing more than external mirrors of internal processes. They are reflections of our personal transformation and should be seen as associations, not causes.

Smoking, for example, symbolizes withdrawal. A person hides behind a smoke screen because of a need to build a barrier between him- or herself and the outside world.

Radiations may also be associations. One is welcome to argue that in the Hiroshima bombing, the correlation between radiation and the subsequent leukemia that many people developed is undeniable. Then again, there are other statistical associations worth considering. One could argue as well for strong light, shock waves, vibration or even the Japanese language as being statistical risk factors, and therefore possible causes in the traditional way of thinking. It is my belief that the intense emotional trauma and the way those individuals dealt with it played a crucial causal part in the development of many cases of leukemia, whereas other effects may have been associations with aggravating effects. In any event, this is food for thought and I don't intend to force a particular way of thinking upon anyone.

BREAST CANCER EXAMPLE: MARY ANNE

Mary Anne is a sweet 46-year-old woman who discovered a lump in her left breast a few days ago. She has always been health conscious, so she sees her doctor for some tests. Unfortunately, her fears become a reality. The tests reveal that she has breast cancer, and that some of her lymph nodes are affected, too. She will probably need treatment. Now let's take a look at the fabric of Mary Anne's life with regard to the symbolic expression of the breasts (nurturing).

Mary Anne comes from a rational, conservative family. Rules were rules and allowance of creativity and its expression were much needed qualities in her family. Some of her family members have had breast cancer also, mirroring the issue for the whole family. Mary Anne was a late child because her mother waited for the right time to have her.

Mary Anne longed for something different than the rationalized expression of love and nurturing. She subconsciously wanted to express her love and nurturing qualities to somebody or something. Unfortunately, she did not have too many dolls in her house and pets were not allowed. Her motherhood instincts had no clear target for a long time; they were suppressed in favor of what her family told her a girl should do in order to succeed in society.

This early psychological shaping influenced all of her relationships. Mary Anne had friends but they were kept at a distance, even though she deeply wanted more affection and close relationships. Over time it became more and more difficult for her to naturally express appreciation, be carefree and joyful. The man she married naturally mirrored her behavior, and soon there was friction in their relationship. She tended to be absorbed with logical considerations, such as the splitting of responsibilities with her husband. Mary Anne wanted him to be there for her more, and she wanted to do the same for him, but her preconditioning prevented her from knowing how to be naturally nurturing. Soon enough, divorce was inevitable.

She was left once again with nobody to nurture. At times she would suffocate people with her attention. Unfortunately, all these feelings and urges were labeled as irrational by Mary Anne and suppressed as much as she could. She started to focus on other aspects of her life and intentionally refused herself the nurturing opportunities life was offering her. She resented her feminine aspects for making her dependent and vulnerable. During this times of emotional abuse, small cancerous cells were born in her left breast. For a while, everything was under control, but her feelings grew harder over time. The more she tried to avoid nurturing in her life, the more opportunities and mirrors were presented to her.

At this point in her life, she discovered the cancerous nodule. The cancer had spread to her lymphatic system, which symbolically carries proteins – life building blocks, plans and projects – to the blood and from there to the whole body. The composition of the lymphatic fluid represents one cell's contribution to the whole body in the same way Mary Anne would feel herself contributing to society by nurturing somebody.

Her lymphatic system was symbolically affected and needed a cleansing. Mary Anne wanted to make a difference by taking care of somebody, but at the same time she suppressed these feelings and never let them flourish in real life. At some point she couldn't accept this condition any longer – the frustrated desire to mother somebody drove her over the edge.

We have to emphasize here that all these processes took place in her subconscious, without her being fully aware of them. She only knew that something was out of control, but couldn't accept things the way they were. Meanwhile, cancer cells mirrored all these conditions.

At her doctor's suggestion Mary Anne finally had surgery and the cancer was removed. Unexpectedly, for the first time in her life, she had something to nurture: her surgery wound and her past affliction with cancer. She had become the center of other people's attention. People were genuinely expressing their concerns and offering support, and she was openly seeking deeper, more trusting communication with them. Her usual, superficial acquaintances with people were being transformed into deep, sincere friendships. The cancer led her to a more natural and loving way of life. She realized that her illness had been a blessing in disguise. After the surgery, Mary Anne's life gradually returned to a normal pattern and, for the first time, she was truly enjoying it.

DEPRESSION

Why is depression becoming a problem of such large proportions in our society? What does it have to do with our lifestyle? How can depression possibly be helpful in our life? The answer to these questions come more or less automatically, once we understand some of the basic mechanisms of this dis-ease.

We'll start with the assumption that depression may be a mental and emotional pattern that befalls certain people during crisis times. It is interesting to note that not all people respond to the same challenges in the same ways: some people feel stuck and become depressed when confronted with a relatively minor upset, while others excel in the face of major challenges. All crises are in fact subjective personal perceptions. One person may not think of a particular situation as something major, but the affected person may experience lack of purpose and see no "light at the end of the tunnel."

Let us suppose that you are in love with someone and he/she breaks up with you. You may be so affected as to commit suicide, but your parents are relieved that you didn't get stuck with this person for life. It is a matter of perception. Some people may go through depressive feelings once in a lifetime, while others experience them over and over. Depression always denotes a time of personal crisis and frustration, where a situation is perceived as a painful, hopeless struggle without purpose. Consequently, the patient lacks motivation and energy.

But how did he/she get to this point? My opinion is that the person did not follow their intuition. They lived by standards that were in conflict with their own sense of right action. Standards are other people's limitations imposed upon us.

At the same time, we are all unique, therefore, all answers to life questions are strictly personal and unique. When we are confused by external standards imposed by others, we tend to ignore the source to all answers, which always lies within. When we do what we love and live with integrity for ourselves, we naturally enjoy the journey. When we follow our calling, everything we do is fun and easy.

It is when we deviate into different standards and ignore our calling, that life begins to feel like a struggle. Things become tough. Confusion and self-judgment will attract difficulties and judgment from other people. Disharmony with ourselves is reflected in the loss of self-confidence and faith.

Dissatisfaction with the past and future block the patient's ability to live in the present. They forget that now is always the point of power. Depression is there to close a road that leads nowhere for an individual. One is most willing to break with the past when frustrated, upset and unhappy. If the person is open to taking a deeper look inside, new solutions will emerge. Depression is a wake-up call – a mechanism designed to take us out of a path that is not ours. Depression is forcing the individual to make a shift and turn off a road that leads nowhere.

A depressed individual always forgets his personal power to change things in life and create new realities. Consequently, depression only appears when one doubts one's ability to affect the future, when one plays the victim and when one does not live up to one's full potential.

We value victims in our society. We give aid, sympathy and assistance. Being a victim is a standard way for many people to receive love and attention that they might not otherwise get. It is not socially acceptable to be self-responsible, but it is respectable to be a victim. Do we ever wonder why there are so many lawyers around?

Depressed people need to realize the cause of their upset and look at their life again. The cause needs to be recognized in order for the condition to be released. Depressed individuals lack energy because most of their energy is consumed by fighting themselves and blocking the best in them. When we do what we love to do in life, we feel enough energy to complete the task easily.

There is always a death of an inner dream that pushes people into depression. The left (logical) prefrontal cortex and the anterior limbic system in the brain (that processes emotions) shut down. This means we stop planning, don't care anymore and become emotionally numb. In a depressed patient, dream activity begins early during the night and lasts longer than in a healthy person. Increased dreaming suggests that there is plenty of processing and perhaps many dream messages that try to convince the individual to follow his love.

These patients have to become aware that is they who created the loss, and they also are the ones able to create happiness again. Nobody else will make them happy again; only they themselves have the power to learn and step ahead.

One can avoid depression by paying attention to early warning signs. When something feels boring or unnatural, our emotional selves give us a clue that we are not following a path that is aligned with our purpose. It may happen that a friend feels great about a path you are considering, but if you are not feeling the same, the path may be theirs, not yours. Let them have their opinion, respect their rights to have an opinion, but follow your love.

DEPRESSION EXAMPLE: SARAH

Let us analyze the case of Sarah, a 22-year-old living at home with her parents. Sarah is going to college and has a part-time job. She is from a well-educated, upper middle class environment. Her parents are expecting her to graduate from college and start a prestigious, well-paying career. All these assumptions have been ingrained in their relationship and act as powerful, unwritten rules.

Sarah accepts this lifestyle and doesn't even think much about it. She thinks this is her path, too, but deep inside Sarah has never come to peace with this lifestyle. She has always been fond of free and creative activities. She sometimes catches herself flipping through travel or leisure magazines or enjoying documentaries.

Her life changes when she meets Greg, a young energetic sales person in town to visit some friends. Sarah is attracted to his unrestricted lifestyle, his extensive travel opportunities, and his fierce sense of independence. Greg doesn't earn very much, but he couldn't care less about it. Notice that Greg is symbolically mirroring Sarah's deeper longing. They instantly fall in love. Sarah feels more energy and fun being around Greg. However, Sarah's parents disapprove of their relationship because of Greg's lifestyle. They want somebody more conventional for their daughter, so Greg and Sarah partially conceal their romance. Greg delays his departure from Sarah's hometown to convince her to come with him. Sarah is faced with a tough decision. She knows she would rather drop college and go with Greg, but she also feels the pressure to stay home, finish college, etc. Her conventional upbringing wins the upper hand and she turns down Greg's offer.

Meanwhile, Sarah's motivation to attend college is vanishing. She is confused. In fact, after Greg leaves she doesn't feel like doing anything. In other words, Sarah is ignoring her dreams and accepting other people's standards. Her actions are perceived by her as a struggle with no purpose. She is losing her appetite (her desire to experience life events even in a symbolic form) and sleeps a lot (refuge into the subconscious). She even has some suicidal thoughts. Sarah stops living in the present and loses all hope and confidence in herself. She feels worthless and unable to change her future. Her parents are extremely concerned but don't understand her behavior. They don't perceive their own standards as limiting and fail to understand that, while these standards may work for them, they are not necessarily right for Sarah.

Sarah subconsciously created this crisis in order to force herself to close the road that leads nowhere for her. The crisis is forcing her to take a deeper look at her life. Yet even at this point her choices are unlimited. Following Greg or staying home are only two among an infinite number of possibilities to choose from. It is up to Sarah to create the right path for herself.

The present is always the point of power. Sarah is a clear case of a reactive depression, but in fact all depressions are reactive to something. People like Sarah need help; they need friends to support them, help them acknowledge their own dreams, and then follow those dreams that energize and fill them with vitality.

ULCERATIONS AND GASTRITIS

Ulcerations and gastritis are similar in their symbolic interpretations. The prevalent issues usually relate to a deeper acceptance of symbolic nourishment. When acceptance of nourishment is compromised, it doesn't nourish or fulfill our deeper longings. As a consequence, we react with a variable inflammatory personal resentment.

Patients with these conditions have difficulty receiving the nourishment joyfully and accepting the bright side of each experience. They are oblivious to the fact that each experience is exactly what we need at any given point in time, even though the deeper meanings might not yet be clear to us. There is often a clinging to old ideas and improper, outdated ways of actions.

These patients also have trouble assimilating and enjoying the benefit and wisdom of each life experience. A patient with duodenal ulcers may be experiencing agitation of the stomach (correlated with increased stomach emptying), whereas a patient with stomach ulcers may experience tension and delayed stomach emptying (correlated with attachment to old experiences). These are all general interpretations and further exploration is necessary. Before we go into those, a review of **Table 9**

	Table 9: Ulcers	
DUODENAL ULCER:	**STOMACH ULCER:**	**GASTRITIS:**
Appears in the 40s	Appears in the 50s	Appears later in adult life
Sharp, deep, penetrating	Deep, penetrating	Diffuse and superficial
Round or oval	Round or oval	Linear, growing along folds
Heals and recurs	Heals and recurs	
Stomach empties rapidly	Stomach emptying delayed	
Pain relieved by food	Pain accentuated by food	

and **Figure 21** for a deeper understanding of the symptoms and symbolism is recommended.

Duodenal Ulcer

The duodenum, which is the first portion of the intestines, represents the transit zone between the stomach and the intestines. Symbolically, it is an action zone where the contents of the stomach, after being accepted, rearranged and digested to a certain stage, are thrown into action.

A typical duodenal ulcer is a sharp, round, penetrating lesion in the first inch of the duodenum. It is surrounded by inflammation and occurs most frequently in males around forty years of age. This type of ulceration is a round (unmanifested) loss of physical substance (lack of physical experience) that is sharply demarcated (clear cut issue) and deep (deeply penetrates the physical, emotional and mental layers of experience). Surrounding this central issue is an inflammation (anger of variable degrees), either acute or chronic (new and intense or long-standing). Ulcerations usually appear at a time when the patient is confronting a specific issue, but if the lesson is not learned, it may recur again and again. If the patient recognizes the problem and takes appropriate steps (appropriate for this

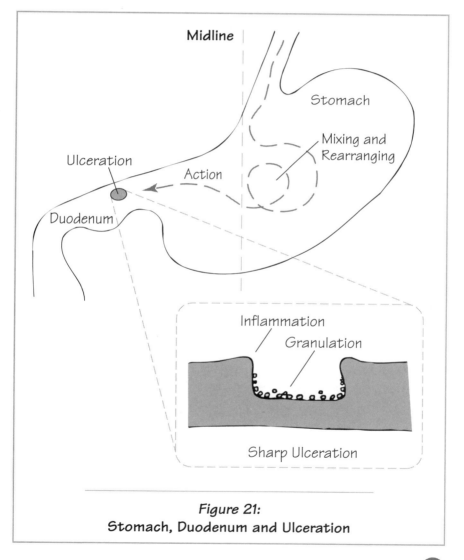

Figure 21:
Stomach, Duodenum and Ulceration

individual only), the ulceration is healed. If the lesson is not learned, the ulceration may reappear months or years later, when a similar challenge arises.

Duodenal ulcers manifest more frequently in males in their forties because this is the time when males have the opportunity to put into logical, constructive action (right side) what they have intuitively accepted and prepared (beliefs) all their lives. The forties is the decade when an individual reaches the peak of their ability to manifest material things in life, as they are no longer in school or under parental guidance, and have accumulated enough life experiences to draw from. In short, this is the time when an individual is most anchored in the physical form.

Ulcer patients exhibit a characteristic lack of genuine, joyful acceptance of new actions and emotions. This frequently translates into pain that is relieved temporarily by eating, especially proteins (proteins can be considered building blocks of life structures, symbolic of our belief system put into action). In other words, ingestion of a surrogate decreases the denial. The issue is usually realized, at least subconsciously, but not acted upon. Food is a symbolic substitute for life experiences that we need. These patients tend to avoid rearranging and rethinking issues. There is usually plenty of action in their life, but this action is not in harmony with their deeper feelings and is not openly accepted. We can understand this pattern better with an example.

DUODENAL ULCER EXAMPLE: STEVE

Our subject is Steve, a 36-year-old male. He has an active life and just got married a year ago. He always searched for some drama in his life, but this need was not consciously acknowledged. This symbolic need for dramatic experiences was reflected in a craving for spicy foods whenever he felt life was too boring.

Long after the honeymoon, Steve feels the need for some spice in his life. Weighing the pros and cons more subconsciously than consciously, he secretly begins to see another woman, Kelly. Their affair grows slowly but steadily.

One day Kelly proposes that Steve move in with her. On this day Steve experiences pain in his stomach for the first time, signaling a serious reaction to that proposal. Steve develops a round ulceration in his duodenum. The ulceration represents issues about some unmanifested (round) action. This action is usually a culmination of previous thoughts, emotions and issues. Duodenal ulcers are related with putting thoughts into action. Steve doesn't feel good about moving in with Kelly, but at the same time he doesn't want to give up their relationship. Soon, Kelly asks him to decide, one way or another. For Steve, there seems to be an impending loss either way he decides. That loss physically manifests into a deep ulceration (which is, in fact, a loss of substance), affecting more than one layer of his duodenum. We can say that Steve has a clear cut problem that is affecting him on different layers – physically, emotionally and mentally.

Steve is angry with himself for being forced to make a decision, and that anger manifests in a moderate degree of inflammation around the ulcer. He is agitated, and consequently his stomach speeds up food processing.

Steve experiences relief from pain whenever he eats. In other words, eating (a substitute for actions) has a soothing effect on his pain. This substitute type of action temporarily eases his indecision, which lasts for several weeks. Finally, he comes to the decision of leaving Kelly. He feels good about this, and his pain subsides. The ulceration eventually heals.

Six months later Steve has a relapse with Kelly. Naturally, his symbolic ulceration reappears, as does the pain. Over the years, Steve's ulcers keep reappearing. For a closer observer, it seems that life events are suggestive of the disease process, and vice versa. A good friend would point that out, and that would be a new start for Steve. The message, once acknowledged, makes the need for the messenger obsolete.

Gastric Ulcers

Gastric ulcers are somewhat similar to duodenal ulcers, but different in location and behavior. Typically they nest themselves in the lower part of the stomach. The upper stomach functions as a holding site, while the lower part mixes and dissolves food in preparation for its passage into the duodenum.

The gastric ulcer patient feels nauseated and in pain. His body has difficulties assimilating and processing food. Symbolically, the patient is having difficulties assimilating and processing life experiences. The gastric location of this ulceration (usually low and in the back) symbolizes rearranging, mixing, dissolving, analyzing and rethinking issues.

The onset of this type of problem is common around age fifty. The ulceration is usually deep, sometimes perforating through the stomach wall and may bleed frequently. A crucial aspect of one's path is desperately asking to be reanalyzed, accepted and reintegrated into personal life. The mortality rate of gastric ulcer patients is higher than that of duodenal ulcer patients, sometimes indicating that the issue is a matter of accepting and growing versus refusing and dying.

The issue is a specific one because the ulceration is well delineated. Its posterior location (in the back) suggests that it relates to a longing for acceptance of life the very way it is. Gastric ulcers occur close to the body's midline, which symbolically represents axial issues for the patient's future growth. Reluctance to reconsider and rethink such an issue is a classic cause of pain.

Laziness in passing the food from the left to the right side of the body denotes obvious difficulties in transforming intuitive, abstract thought forms into logical, concrete thinking. The obstacle in the transition from abstract to concrete thinking causes delay in the transportation of food through the stomach exit. This explains the difference between gastric ulcers, characterized by delayed emptying of stomach contents, and duodenal ulcers, characterized by hastened stomach emptying.

Gastritis

In gastritis, a large part of the stomach lining is affected by diffuse inflammation. The corresponding symbolic issue is generalized rather than specific, and involves a wide range of life issues. Inflammation signifies anger. The superficial physical discomfort indicates that the patient is only minimally affected by these issues (they are not life and death issues).

It is interesting to note that the inflammation follows the linear folds of the stomach. This tells us that the anger is aimed at directional lines that the patient chooses. The inflammatory reaction can be the result of acutely stressful events, such as severe trauma, major surgery, shock, massive burns or severe infections. If this is the case, the reaction is accompanied by swelling (clinging to emotions), erosion and friability of the stomach lining (acceptance of the physical condition is disintegrating) and bleeding (life force and energy are leaking).

Gastritis can also be a slow, chronic process that frequently leads to a slow working stomach. This condition usually affects the elderly and those who are not having an easy time accepting and enjoying their lives. Glands, which are secreting different fluids that correspond to specific emotions, also decrease in number and activity as we get older.

Gastritis patients are frequently experiencing difficulty absorbing Vitamin B_{12} (twelve is the number of completion, signifying completion of the spiritual path). Vitamin B_{12} contains cobalt (an element with spiritual significance, indigo/violet in color) which plays a role similar to iron in living processes. When

Vitamin B_{12} is not properly absorbed, DNA formation is impaired (our genetic blueprint for life loses clarity). The equilibrium between DNA and RNA is disturbed. Symbolically, we can say that there is more RNA (the way we act in life) and less DNA (our genetic blueprint of life in its perfect state) in the cells, indicating that we have deviated from our life purpose. Our spiritual purpose becomes obscured and completion of our path is stalled. The consequences are anemia (lack of vitality and energy), reluctance to accept events (malabsorption and gastritis) and neurological changes (feeling out of control, refusal to perceive the higher, cosmic significance of an experience).

Pneumonia and Lung Disease

Our lungs are one of the most spiritual organs of the body because they take in oxygen, the spark of life. Oxygen is the origin of fire (literally and symbolically) and has the power to keep alive every cell, to activate the primal life force, lift depression and bring vitality to mind and body. The act of breathing represents the process of taking in and giving out. Our breath reveals much about the way we accept or deny life experiences. For more details of the symbolic significance of the lungs and respiratory system, please refer to **Part II**, *The Respiratory Network: Lungs/Large Intestine.*

Air is absorbed into the lungs by a tree-like branching system that symbolically represents the tree of life. The fact that there is a left and right lung symbolizes cooperation and duality. Duality is represented by the number two, which contains the power of multiplication, and which expresses itself in the branching concept. Each lung is comprised of ten segments, each one with its own individual ventilation and circulation. The number ten, again, symbolizes oneness of the individual with the universal. The right lung (masculine side, symbolized by the number "3") has three lobes and the left (feminine side, symbolized by the number "2") has two lobes. Together, they add up to five, the number of life.

Each lobe further divides into lobules and segments which are arranged in the same pattern of geometric figures that can be observed in the bones and elsewhere: the triangle, the circle and the square (or rectangle).

The lungs look like triangles whose bases are situated above the diaphragm. The diaphragm is a muscle that demarcates a borderline between the abdomen (the more primitive animalic and physical part of us) and the thorax (a more refined, spiritual place). Periodically, the diaphragm oscillates upward and downward. This symbolically indicates the extent of our tendency to accept physical and spiritual guidance at any given moment (see **Figure 22**). Ideally, there is a state of dynamic balance between these two essential components of our beings.

When the bases of the lungs are more ventilated than the upper portions, this implies that we receive energy and guidance mostly with respect to the coarse, three-dimensional physical realm. Women tend to be more receptive to spiritual guidance than men, which explains why they naturally breathe more into the upper portion of the lungs. This general statement is, of course, all a matter of degree. Both men and women breathe with lower and upper lungs at the same time.

The way we receive air is a measure of our openness. This is even reflected in the language: when we are shocked or upset we hold our breath. The word inspiration is related to inhalation; the term is a symbolic expression of our openness to accept higher (divine) guidance. Exhalation measures our capacity to be involved in the physical realm, to contract, to end cycles and to express ourselves. We accept inspiration through inhalation and respond back to nature through exhalation.

Asthma

In asthma, exhalation is partially blocked and the inhaled air is retained inside the lungs. The lungs show inflammation (anger) symbolically directed toward the exhaling process. Parallel to this obstacle in physical expression, one can usually observe a stifling of the speech, which is a symbolic form of expression. This is because in order to speak, one needs to exhale. Individuals affected by this disease have a difficult time expressing themselves fully; they have difficulties manifesting in the physicality. They tend to be uncomfortable in the physical reality and long to become more of what they truly are (divine beings).

This might explain why children are most frequently affected by this condition. Asthma in children usually improves over time as they get used to the physical aspect of the human condition.

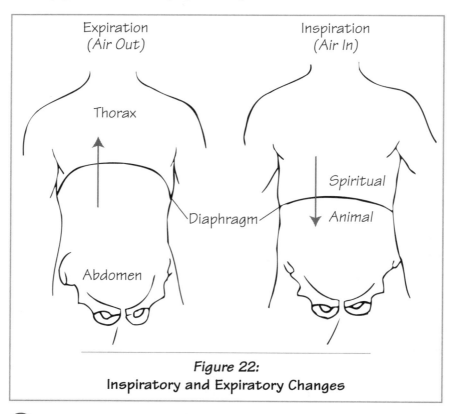

Figure 22:
Inspiratory and Expiratory Changes

Symptoms of asthma may include spasms of bronchial muscles, swelling, secretions and inflammation, all of which represent a reluctance to act and accept. Coughing and expectoration generally symbolize an unwillingness to accept. Serious emotional expressions of this refusal to accept (anger and violent reactions of suffocation) may overwhelm the patient. The world is not experienced as a safe place to express oneself. Yet, various stimuli that trigger asthma attacks are always symbolic reminders of the patient's physicality: dust, pollution, exercise, occupational factors, stress, etc. The majority of asthma attacks are brief, but they may be serious for the patient.

Life progresses in cycles, such as day/night, etc. When we block one part of a cycle, in this case exhalation, the other part of the cycle (chest expansion and inhalation) becomes also obstructed. In this way, new inspiration and guidance is not physically possible until harmony is restored.

It is no coincidence that many asthma attacks strike while the patient is dreaming. Asthma attacks that occur while the patient is dreaming (not just sleeping) were discussed in the chapter of cluster headaches. The attack is a reaction to the message contained in the dreams.

Tuberculosis

Different diseases of the lungs are characterized by different patterns which are all unique in their symbolic meaning. Tuberculosis, for example, operates on a low level of intensity. The unique trait of a tuberculosis patient is their perception that they are being forced to live in some form of confinement. Frequently, they are socially deprived and have a low standard of living. This is again a reflection of their perception and not necessarily the actual reality. The chronic (long-term) preoccupation with this issue of confinement can become quite consuming; tuberculosis is, in fact, a disease of consumption. Symbolically, the lungs become consumed inside a cavernous process which is confining those changes. The lesson associated with tuberculosis is a long, slow process of integrating the seemingly confined human existence with one's unbounded spiritual nature.

Pneumonia

Pneumonia is a lung inflammation. Not surprisingly, it still continues to be a leading cause of death, particularly in children and the elderly. A pneumonia patient symbolically refuses to breathe with the part of the lung that is affected. This disease is a symbolic refusal to take in life, to take up space and to exist. Emotional wounds are intense. The patient tends to be depressed, desperate and tired of living. He or she may even feel that life is not worth living anymore under the present circumstances. In some cases, pneumonia becomes a quick method to pass away. Is it still a mystery now why so many long-term hospitalized elderly patients contract pneumonia? Mortality for pneumonia has not changed much with modern medical advances, probably because of the profound meaning of this disease – a strong, sometimes desperate desire to give up life.

A pneumonia patient is usually angered toward a part of his inspiration and symbolically closes down the lung territory that is concerned with it. Pneumonia is triggered by a major upset within an individual's life. The patient's generalized fever may indicate anger toward spiritual inspiration, symbolized by inhalation. Each breath brings painful sensations (denials). The patient may experience chills (refusal to be in the present moment; desire to escape from life experiences). A persistent cough may indicate rejection of guidance, ideas or life situations that trigger the disease process. Local inflammation quickly develops in the affected part of the lung.

When a person experiences an event as disturbing (for example, a small cut or scratch), the body responds by producing local substances which increase and speed up its natural healing process. In the case of pneumonia, this increased substance flow (increased permeability) allows fluids (emotions) to flood the pulmonary alveoli (small sacs which the lungs are made of). The liquid contents of these sacs is then changed by enzymes into a solid substance. The affected part of

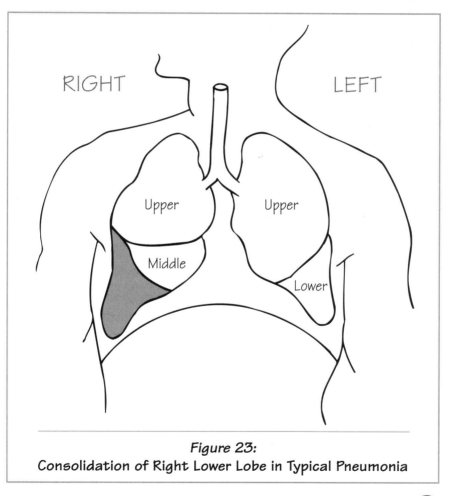

Figure 23:
Consolidation of Right Lower Lobe in Typical Pneumonia

the lung then contains solid matter, which prevents oxygen from reaching the site. The fact that these fluids solidify into solid physical matter signifies that the corresponding emotional issues desperately want to be addressed and are becoming more and more prevalent in order to be noticed.

Why is this happening? Generally, emotions that are not addressed tend to solidify into physical matter, which is a physical mirror of our emotional states. This consolidation in the lung that we encounter in pneumonia, has many symbolic implications. For example, if oxygen cannot reach the right lower lobe, this affliction may be considered as a symbolic refusal to accept the masculine or logical part of a physical problem (see **Figure 23**).

Pneumonia usually resolves in a matter of days because the symbolic cause is acute. Patients either resolve their issues and restart to breathe or choose to move on and die. They are not victims of anything. All aspects of our environment, including bacteria and viruses, are nothing other than symbolic reflections of our attitudes, be they external or internal. From this perspective, even aggressive bacteria can help us. All we need to do is be open to their message (see pages 92 through 96).

Pneumonia Example:
Bob

Let us consider Bob, a 36-year old, working hard, but earning just enough to make ends meet. He is now working overtime and weekends, hoping to get ahead financially.

Bob was married once and has three children. His wife left him three years ago, taking two of the children with her. Bob still has Nicky, a sweet six-year old boy. They get along well, but it is hard for Bob to raise Nicky the way he would like to. Bob is working more and more hours while Nicky spends most of his time in day care. However, Bob is determined not to give up, even under extreme pressure and responsibility. Things go well, until one unfortunate day when little Nicky breaks his leg and is forced to stay home from school. Bob has to spend more time with him, but is also facing many medical bills. The logical solution seems to be to work even harder.

Bob's body finally reaches a limit; he responds by feeling extremely tired, starts coughing, and catches a flu. But soon another element adds to this inner conflict of having to work hard versus wanting to be with Nicky. Nicky's mother hears about the situation and files a lawsuit to take Nicky away.

This is the straw that breaks the camel's back. Bob feels exhausted and desperate; it seems as though all the world is against him. He is developing fever (anger) and chills (he symbolically wants to escape the situation). Bob subconsciously stops breathing with the lower part of his right lung (he refuses to understand the reasoning behind this concrete, physical situation). His breathing is becoming rapid and shallow (he refuses to fully accept life). Soon after this, there is pain (denial) when breathing in that area of his lungs.

Bob is now coughing vigorously, bringing up rusty colored (blood tinged) sputum. Symbolically, emotions and joy of life are being rejected. He is grunting with each exhalation – a deep sound correlated with difficulties in letting go. Bob's lips and nails are turning blue: a symbolic inability to handle a situation (nails) and express himself (lips). The difficulty with self-expression is further symbolized by a herpetic eruption on the corner of his mouth. He is being invaded by thoughts and words that needed to erupt, but had been denied; as a result they are being perceived as painful. Bob is feeling angry and overloaded at having to process all these events at once, so his liver starts to deteriorate. Fluids (emotions) are flooding his lower right lung. These emotions are beginning to consolidate in his lungs (they are becoming a threatening physical reality for Bob). The involved part of the lung is turning gray. Gray symbolically implies that Bob does not want to be involved in these experiences. Strands of fibrin (symbolic of solid, rigid consequences), leukocytes (acute spiritual help) and red blood cells (vitality, small amounts of oxygen) are leaking into the affected area.

Numerous bacteria are also present, highly representative of Bob's emotional experience. These bacteria (*pneumococci*) are lancet shaped with a thick capsule around them, and are arranged in groups of two (see **Figure 24**). Nicky is the only thing left for Bob and he is building a thick, symbolic wall around themselves; it is now him and Nicky against the whole world. They are fighting an external condition with a symbolic lancet shape. This behavior (bacteria) consumes Bob's vitality (hemolysis or destroyed blood is present around that area).

This particular species of bacteria is part of our normal behavior, but usually they occur in much milder conditions and lack the desperate wall around them. Under normal circumstances these bacteria symbolize Bob's care of Nicky (or anybody else), but this has now been intensified into an extreme defense reaction.

Bob is very sick for three days in a row. His ex-wife is visiting him at the hospital. She is impressed by his suffering and is helping him and Nicky as best she can. Touched by their bond and struggles, she finally decides not to pursue her lawsuit.

The next day, as if by a miracle, Bob is breathing better and starting to recover. Bacteria are being eliminated one by one as the healing process takes over. In fact, as the defensive behavior disappears, bacteria are symbolically losing their walls and being eaten away by various cells until they have disappeared from the lungs. The new sensation of freedom is sudden, and in a matter of hours, Bob is feeling much better. He is starting to breathe

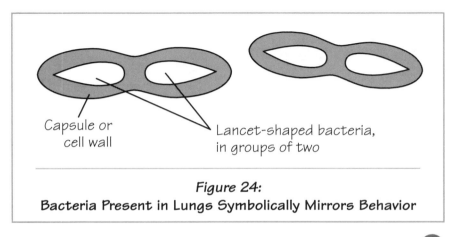

Capsule or cell wall

Lancet-shaped bacteria, in groups of two

Figure 24:
Bacteria Present in Lungs Symbolically Mirrors Behavior

again with his right lower lung. The consolidation has disappeared. His fever is subsiding and Bob is on his way to recovery.

A new level of acceptance and gratitude has come into Bob's life. The joy of everyday living, the inspiration of his son and the acceptance of everyday experiences found a new meaning for Bob. His story and others are repeated every day, thousands of times. Each one has its own particular details and problems. Each one is cry for a new awareness. In many cases, this new awareness comes to the forefront of our daily experiences, opening new horizons and possibilities. If this happens, the illness fulfills its purpose and leaves peacefully.

It is my hope that many will start to become more and more receptive to these symbolic messages and will listen to their inner healing desire. *Healing takes place from within the self, by changing one's belief structure.*

❖ ❖ ❖

Afterword
Sources
Symbolic Interpretation
Index

❖ ❖ ❖

AFTERWORD

This book is an opportunity for self-discovery, intended to help people connect to a deeper level within themselves. This deeper level is a place of great wisdom and healing power in all of us.

You, the reader, will take from this book whatever you need on your path. You may read and be interested in two lines, three chapters or the whole book. Trust that what doesn't resonate with you is not for your best unfoldment in the way your subconscious has designed it. You might find it helpful to pay special attention to what stirs or challenges you. Observe your reactions and notice any resistance. There you might find the key to your unique truth.

Trust that the truth is changing. Allow yourself to grow. Trust that scientific research is not advanced enough to prove everything, because science innocently mirrors the present focus of society. When the focus or the color of the eyeglasses changes, the scientific reality will change with it. It may take 200 years to prove all these concepts, and it will happen only if we collectively accept them.

The only way to understand anything new is by allowing this new concept to connect with us on a sincere, deep level. If we do this, we take the first step toward connecting with our multi-dimensional divine self. In fact, everything around is just a small mirror of this multidimensional divine self.

This book was designed for you to understand the process of disease on a deeper level. No deeper scientific explanations are given, but if you read the book up to this point, you did not need them. Your heart knows what is true for you and does not need scientific explanations.

Notice also that no attempts were made in this book to cover treatments or healing techniques. They will probably be covered in other books to come. There is no better way to healing, or indeed to anything; solutions to problems are unique and personal. This is why I believe quick tips are to be avoided. Everything is ultimately up to you, the reader. Only you have the answers – all the answers. Time has come to allow the answers to speak; all you need to do is listen.

Last but not least, let's remember that the disease symbolism mentioned in this book have only general validity. A personal perspective and interpretation is not only recommended, but necessary in each case.

Once again, I express my acknowledgment and respect to all beings and wish you fun and delight in healing yourself. Remember that when the focus changes, reality will change.

SOURCES

Significant Bibliography:

1. *Spirit Speaks;* Magazine Collection, Tucson, AZ.

2. *Harrison's Principles of Internal Medicine;* J. Wilson, E. Braumwald.

3. *You Can Heal Your Life;* Louise Hay.

4. *Between Heaven and Earth: A Guide to Chinese Medicine;* H. Beinfield, E. Korngold.

5. *Sacred Geometry;* Robert Lawlor.

6. *Light Emerging;* Barbara Ann Brennan.

7. *The Matter Myth;* Paul Davies and John Gribbin.

8. **Chart 1**: "Five Phase Correspondences" reprinted by permission from *The Five Phases of Food;* John W. Garvy, Jr. (*Wellbeing Books;* phone: 617/969-9711).

9. *Conversations with God – An Uncommon Dialogue;* Neale Donald Walsch.

10. *God I Am – From Tragic to Magic;* Peter O. Erbe.

11. *Searching for Light: Michael's Information for a Time of Change;* Carol Heidemann (*Twelve Star Publishing;* phone: 301/473-9035).

12. *Prelude to Ascension;* Janet McClure and Vywamus (*Light Technology Publishing*).

Quotes & Mottos:

Book Motto   *Spirit Speaks* Magazine.

Part I   *Searching for Light;* Carol Heidemann (p. 198).

Part II   *The Bible* (Matthew).

Parts III & IV   I admit to having forgotten the source, but give thanks.

Part V   *Prelude to Ascension;* Janet McClure and Vywamus, (p. 619).

Symbol Interpretation

Personal Interpretations of Some of this Book's Symbols (limited to one or several meanings)

A:

Abdomen: primal force, basic instincts.

Abscess: contained anger & destruction.

Accidents: rebellion, hurting inside.

Acne: occasional dislike, anger about self-image.

Adrenal glands: being involved, caring, persevering.

Air: mental element & qualities.

Anemia: lack of joy & vitality.

Anger: upset about an unexpected outcome.

Ankles: stability & support, flexibility of direction in new activities.

Anorexia: rejection of life experiences.

Antibodies: elements of defense.

Arms:
    left arm: love.
    right arm: wisdom.

Arteries: pathways of life.

Arthritis: criticism, inflexibility.

Atherosclerosis: narrow ways of life, rigid ways of being.

Assimilation: acceptance.

Asthma: rejection of physicality.

Autonomic neuropathy: relationship issues.

B:

Back: receptivity, support, the past.
    lower back: (sacred) support.
Back problems: lack of support & receptivity.
Backside headaches: denial of the process of acknowledging
    what we see.
Bacteria: primitive, defensive elements that mirror our behavior.
Belching: rejection of mental & emotional experiences.
Bladder: emotional control, holding on.
Bladder problems: holding on to emotions.
Bleeding: leaking of joy.
Blood: joy, vitality, nourishment, vital force.
Blood problems: lack of satisfaction & enjoyment.
Blood congestion: emotional hang-up, stagnation of joy.
Bones: stability, firmness, divine support structures.
Bowel problems: difficulty of letting go.
Brain: control, coordination, administrative center.
Breasts: caring, nurturing focus.
Breast problems: problems with nurturing, nourishment.
Breath: ability to expand, take in, live.
Bursitis: anger toward a possibility.

C:

Cancer: being out of control.
Cancerous cells: thoughts of resentment that are out of control.

Cell (normal): normal thought pattern, way of life.

Children: symbolic creations.

Chills: desire to shake off an experience.

Chocolate: indulgence, pleasure, physical sex.

Circle: unmanifest, infinite potential.

Cold: feeling overwhelmed by stress.

Colitis: anger toward letting go.

Colon: issues of elimination, letting go.

Colors:
> **red:** physical energy, dynamism, will, action, vital force;
> **red/orange:** sexual energy;
> **yellow:** expansion, intellect, active intelligence;
> **green:** balancing, healing, growth;
> **blue:** expression, teaching, love, wisdom;
> **violet/indigo:** profound spirituality, transformation;
> **gray:** noninvolvement, neutrality;
> **black:** regeneration, nonparticipation;
> **white:** truth, oneness;
> **silver:** communication;
> **gold:** divinity, Christ consciousness.

Coma: wanting to pass away.

Confusion: refusal to accept & focus.

Connective tissue: active use of divine plan.

Constipation: reluctance to give away, hard to let go.

Coronary thrombosis: blockage of love & joy.

Coughing: rejecting a message.

Cramps: holding, denying.

Craving: signal for a need of balance.

Cysts: trapped emotions.

D:

Deep breathing: acceptance.

Depression: extreme perception of victimhood.

Diabetes: refusal to accept sweetness.

Digestion: assimilation of life experiences.

Diarrhea: running from an emotion, letting go easily.

Dizziness: refusal to focus.

DNA: symbolic blueprint of our destiny.

Downward: stability, strength, support.

E:

Ears: capacity to listen & surrender.

Ear problems: resistance to emotional messages.

Edema: emotional clinging.

Elbows: flexibility in giving.

Emphysema: belief that not much can change.

Enzymes: catalysts of change.

Epilepsy: rejection of life.

Eczema: anger at being seen.

Eyes: insight, capacity to see connections.

Eye problems: refusal to see harmony.

F:

Face: symbolic of facing issues.

Fainting: refusal of an experience.

Fat: protection, insulation.

Fatigue: refusal to participate, to follow true path.

Feet: foundation, basic beliefs, balance, support, understanding.

Feet problems: hurt while stepping forward in life.

Fear: issue with control & letting go.

Female problems: refusing feminine issues.

Feminine: receptivity, intuition, creation.

Fever: generalized anger.

Fingernails: growing focus.

Fingers: focus, details of how issues are handled;
    thumb: stomach/spleen/pancreas;
    index: lungs/large intestine;
    middle: liver/gallbladder;
    ring: kidney/bladder;
    pinky: heart/small intestine.

Fire: spiritual spark.

Focusing: converging of energy.

Food: symbolic of life experiences.

Forehead: foresight, vision.

Fractures: crashing of support structures.

Front: future, qualities of giving.

G:

Gallbladder: balanced timing & planning of actions, discrimination & discernment.

Gas/air: mental element.

Gastritis: anger toward acceptance.

Glands: production of emotions.

Gonads: sexual identity.

H:

Hair: thoughts.

Hands: handling, dealing, taking in, grasping.

Head: control, coordination, truth.

Headaches: confrontations, denial of control issues.

Hearing problems: resistance to emotional messages.

Heart: receiver & transmitter of love & joy.

Heart attack: refusal to (give) love.

Hemorrhage: leaking of joy & vitality.

Hepatitis: anger toward processing.

High blood pressure: high emotional pressure.

Hips: acceptance & flexibility, connecting divine guidance
with individual path.

Hip problems: problems with assimilation/elimination.

Hydrogen: mental element.

Hypertension: refusal to address a conflict, refuge in "busy"-ness.

I:

Ice cream: need to cool down sweet cravings.

Illness: communication being forced.

Imagination: awareness focused on different realities.

Immune system: enthusiasm for life.

Infection: anger, defensive behavior.

Inflammation: anger.

Intestines:
  large intestine: preparation for letting go, giving;
  small intestine: analysis, discrimination;

J:

Joints: flexibility.

Joint capsules: physical limits of symbolic movement.

Joint problems: lack of flexibility.

K:

Kidneys: filters of the emotional flow of life.

Kidney problems: rejection of the flow, deep fear.

Knees: humility, flexibility toward divine will, detachment, letting go.

L:

Laryngitis: anger at one's speech & self-expression.

Left side: feminine, qualities of receptivity, creativity, intuition.

Legs (lower extremities including hip joint):
    left leg: goodness, virtue;
    right leg: justice.

Liquid: emotional element.

Liver: organ of purification, action, processing, integration.

Liver problems: refusal to process, act.

Love: unity, connection, harmony, God.

Lungs: freedom, rhythm, harmony, taking in life.

Lymph problems: deep need to cleanse the system of emotional & mental toxins.

M:

Masculine: giving, logical, constructive.

Migraines: resistance to an experience.

Motor neuropathy: (perception of) feeling out of control.

Mouth: taking in nourishment, acceptance.

Muscles: actions, mobility, activity.

Myopia: refusal to see far in the future.

N:

Nails: aggression.

Nausea: rejection of the physical experience.

Neck: connecting link with creative manifestation.

Neck problems: lack of mental expressive flexibility.

Nerves: controlling mechanisms.

Nose: pride.

Numbers:
>**0:** infinite knowledge & mental potential;
>**1:** unity, individuality, beginning;
>**2:** duality, multiplicity, feminine, cooperation;
>**3:** trinity, masculine, energetic, active, self-expression;
>**4:** practicality, organization, materialization;
>**5:** life experiences, freedom;
>**6:** responsibility, work, service;
>**7:** wisdom;
>**8:** accomplishments;
>**9:** compassion, humanitarianism;
>**10:** union of individuality with infinity, path to God;
>**11:** inspiration;

12: completion;

22: universality.

Numbness: refusal to feel.

O:

Obesity: self-protection & insulation.

Osteoarthritis: criticism, stiffness, narrow standards.

Osteophytes: physical restrictions of freedom & choices.

Ovaries: divine possibilities.

Oxygen: spiritual force, spark of life.

P:

Pain: refusal, denial of an experience.

Pancreas: deep acceptance of life events.

Pink: love.

Pituitary: coordination.

Pneumonia: desperate refusal to live.

Prostate problems: sexual regrets, sexual issues of letting go.

Proteins: building blocks.

R:

Right side: masculine qualities of giving, logic, construction.

Right thumb: logic, intellect.

RNA: our way of carrying out our destiny.

S:

Sacral area: creation, sex.

Secretions: emotional reactions.

Sensory neuropathy: refusal to feel.

Short, sharp pain: short, sharp denial.

Shoulders: flexibility, processing, transformations.

Skin: facade, delineations, contact.

Skin problems: issues with self-image.

Slipped disc: slipped support condition.

Small intestines: acceptance of physical experiences.

Smoking: hiding behind a smoke screen.

Solar plexus: emotional center.

Solid: physical.

Sore throat: anger for not expressing oneself.

Spinal column: fundamental support, belief system.

Sprains: anger, reactions toward outrageous movements.

Spring: new beginnings, building up.

Stiffness: rigid philosophy & lifestyle.

Stomach: acceptance, assimilation, receptivity.

Stomach problems: difficulty accepting nourishment & life, unwillingness to accept conflict.

Stroke: lack of joy, blockage of normal functions.

Stuffy nose: reaction to an overwhelming life experience.

Sugars & sweets: sweetness in life.

Swallowing: accepting new experiences.

T:

Taste: symbolic predigestion.

Thorax: spiritual force.

Throat: communication, expression.

Throat problems: problems with expression.

Thymus: innocence, enjoyment.

Thyroid: rhythm & balance, creative control.

Toes: specific focus within core beliefs, specific beliefs.

Tongue: expression, speech.

Tuberculosis: reaction to a belief of having to live in confined conditions.

U:

Ulcers: refusal to accept a loss.

Upward: opening, expressing, communicating.

Uterus: home, nurturing, mother.

V:

Vanilla: family.

Vertebrae:
    C6: ability to feel gratitude;
    C7: ability to think logically;
    L_5-S_1: where physicality meets sacredness.

Viruses: thought patterns.

Vision: physical reflection of beliefs.

Vitamins: catalysts of different processes;
    Vitamin A: purification, protection, beliefs;
    Vitamin B$_1$: assertion of one's unique, individual existence;
    Vitamin B$_2$: the way we process & duplicate;
    Vitamin B$_6$: the way we handle situations;
    Vitamin B$_{12}$: completion of a spiritual path;
    Vitamin C: genuine joy, acceptance of a way of being;
    Vitamin D: deep support of one's beliefs;
    Vitamin E: acceptance of life, change, staying young.

W:

Water: emotions.

White: truth, oneness.

Worry: trying to accept something over & over.

Wind: action, movement.

Wrists: flexibility, acceptance.

INDEX

C:

D:

E:

F:

G:

H:

S:

W:

Y:

Z:

If you have suggestions, want to hear from us
in the future, or would like to be placed on a mailing list
for future events, newsletters, books or clubs related
to this subject, please contact us by email at:

symbols@mailexcite.com

ADDITIONAL TITLES
BY SUNSTAR PUBLISHING LTD.

The Name Book by Pierre Le Rouzic
  ISBN 0-9638502-1-0 $15.95
Numerology/Philosophy. International bestseller. Over 9,000 names with stunningly accurate descriptions of character and personality. How the sound of your name effects who you grow up to be.

Every Day A Miracle Happens by Rodney Charles
  ISBN 0-9638502-0-2 $17.95
Religious bestseller. 365 stories of miracles, both modern and historic, each associated with a day of the year. Universal calendar. Western religion.

Of War & Weddings by Jerry Yellin
  ISBN 0-9638502-5-3 $17.95
History/Religion. A moving and compelling autobiography of bitter wartime enemies who found peace through their children's marriage. Japanese history and religion.

Your Star Child by Mary Mayhew
  ISBN 0-9638502-2-9 $16.95
East/West philosophy. Combines Eastern philosophy with the birthing techniques of modern medicine, from preconception to parenting young adults.

Lighter Than Air by Rodney Charles and Anna Jordan
  ISBN 0-9638502-7-X $14.95
East/West philosophy. Historic accounts of saints, sages and holy people who possessed the ability of unaided human flight.

Bringing Home the Sushi by Mark Meers
  ISBN 1-887472-05-3 $21.95
Japanese philosophy and culture. Adventurous account of of an American businessman and his family living in '90s Japan.

Miracle of Names by Clayne Conings
  ISBN 1-887472-03-7 $13.95
Numerology and Eastern philosophy. Educational and enlightening – discover the hidden meanings and potential of names through numerology.

Voice for the Planet by Anna Maria Gallo
  ISBN 1-887472-00-2 $10.95
Religion/Ecology. This book explores the ecological practicality of native American practices.

Making $$$ At Home by Darla Sims
  ISBN 1-887472-02-9 $25.00
Reference. Labor-saving directory that guides you through the process of making contacts to create a business at home.

Gabriel & the Remarkable Pebbles by Carol Hovin
  ISBN 1-887472-06-1 $12.95
Children/Ecology. A lighthearted, easy-to-read fable that educates children in understanding ecological balances.

Searching for Camelot by Edith Thomas
  ISBN 1-887472-08-8 $12.95
East/West philosophy. Short easy-to-read, autobiographical adventure full of inspirational life lessons.

The Revelations of Ho by Dr. James Weldon
  ISBN 1-887472-09-6 $17.95
Eastern philosophy. A vivid and detailed account of the path of a modern-day seeker of enlightenment.

The Formula by Dr. Vernon Sylvest
  ISBN 1-887472-10-X $21.95
Eastern philosophy/Medical research. This book demystifies the gap between medicine and mysticism, offering a ground breaking perspective on health as seen through the eyes of an eminent pathologist.

Jewel of the Lotus by Bodhi Avinasha
   ISBN 1-887472-11-8 $15.95

Eastern philosophy. Tantric Path to higher consciousness. Learn to increase your energy level, heal and rejuvenate yourself through devotional relationships.

Elementary, My Dear by Tree Stevens
   ISBN 1-887472-12-6 $17.95

Cooking/Health. Step-by-step, health-conscious cookbook for the beginner. Includes hundreds of time-saving menus.

Directory of New Age & Alternative Publications by Darla Sims
   ISBN 1-887472-18-5 $23.95

Reference. Comprehensive listing of publications, events, organizations arranged alphabetically, by category and by location.

Educating Your Star Child by Ed & Mary Mayhew
   ISBN 1-887472-17-7 $16.95

East/West philosophy. How to parent children to be smarter, wiser and happier, using internationally acclaimed mind-body intelligence techniques.

How to be Totally Unhappy in a Peaceful World by Gil Friedman
   ISBN 1-887472-13-4 $11.95

Humor/Self-help. Everything you ever wanted to know about being unhappy: A complete manual with rules, exercises, a midterm and final exam. (Paper.)

No Justice by Chris Raymondo
   ISBN 1-887472-14-2 $23.95

Adventure. Based on a true story, this adventure novel provides behind the scenes insight into CIA and drug cartel operations. One of the best suspense novels of the '90s. (Cloth.)

On Wings of Light by Ronna Herman
   ISBN 1-887472-19-3 $19.95

New Age. Ronna Herman documents the profoundly moving and inspirational messages for her beloved Archangel Michael.

The Global Oracle by Edward Tarabilda & Doug Grimes
ISBN 1-887472-22-3 $17.95

East/West Philosophy. A guide to the study of archetypes, with an excellent introduction to holistic living. Use this remarkable oracle for meditation, play or an aid in decision making.

Destiny by Sylvia Clute
ISBN 1-887472-21-5 $21.95

East/West philosophy. A brilliant metaphysical mystery novel (with the ghost of George Washington) based on A Course In Miracles.

The Husband's Manual by A. & T. Murphy
ISBN 0-9632336-4-5 $9.00

Self-help/Men's Issues. At last! Instructions for men on what to do and when to do it. The Husband's Manual can help a man create a satisfying, successful marriage – one he can take pride in, not just be resigned to.

Cosmic Perspective by Harold Allen
ISBN 1-887472-23-1 $21.95

Science/Eastern philosophy. Eminent cosmologist Harold Allen disproves the "Big Bang Theory" and paves the way for the new era of "Consciousness Theory."

Twin Galaxies Pinball Book of World Records by Walter Day
ISBN 1-887472-25-8 $12.95

Reference. The official reference book for all Video Game and Pinball Players – this book coordinates an international schedule of tournaments that players can compete in to gain entrance into this record book.

How to Have a Meaningful Relationship with Your Computer
by Sandy Berger
ISBN 1-887472-36-3 $18.95

Computer/Self-help. A simple yet amusing guide to buying and using a computer, for beginners as well as those who need a little more encouragement.

The Face on Mars by Harold Allen
  ISBN 1-887472-27-4 $14.95

Science/Fiction. A metaphysical/scientific novel based on the NASA space expedition to Mars.

The Spiritual Warrior by Shakura Rei
  ISBN 1-887472-28-2 $17.95

Eastern philosophy. An exposition of the spiritual techniques and practices of Eastern Philosophy.

The Pillar of Celestial Fire by Robert Cox
  ISBN 1-887472-30-4 $18.95

Eastern philosophy. The ancient cycles of time, the sacred alchemical science and the new golden age.

The Tenth Man by Wei Wu Wei
  ISBN 1-887472-31-2 $15.95

Eastern philosophy. Discourses on Vedanta – the final stroke of enlightenment.

Open Secret by Wei Wu Wei
  ISBN 1-887472-32-0 $14.95

Eastern philosophy. Discourses on Vedanta – the final stroke of enlightenment.

All Else is Bondage by Wei Wu Wei
  ISBN 1-887472-34-7 $16.95

Eastern philosophy. Discourses on Vedanta – the final stroke of enlightenment.

PUBLISHING AND DISTRIBUTING YOUR BOOK IS THIS SIMPLE ...

1. Send us your completed manuscript.
2. We'll review it. Then after acceptance we'll:
   - Register your book with The Library of Congress, Books in Print, and acquire International Standard Book Numbers, including UPC Bar Codes.
   - Design and print your book cover.
   - Format and produce 50 review copies.
   - Deliver review copies (with sales aids) to 20 of the nation's leading distributors and 50 major newspaper, magazine, television and radio book reviewers in the USA and Canada.
   - Organize author interviews and book reviews.
3. Once we have generated pre-orders for 1000 books, New Author Enterprises will enter into an exclusive publishing contract offering up to 50% profit-sharing terms with the author.

PEOPLE ARE TALKING ABOUT US ...

"I recommend New Author Enterprises to any new author. The start-up cost to publish my book exceeded $20,000 – making it nearly impossible for me to do it on my own. New Author Enterprises' ingenious marketing ideas and their network of distributors allowed me to reach my goals for less than $4,000. Once my book reached the distributors and orders started coming in, New Author Enterprises handled everything – financing, printing, fulfillment, marketing – and I earned more than I could have with any other publisher."

— **Rodney Charles,** *best-selling author of Every Day A Miracle Happens*

PUBLISH IT NOW!

116 North Court St., Fairfield IA 52556 • (800) 532-4734
http://www.newagepage.com